VIKING SWORD AND SHIELD FIGHTING

A Step-by-Step Book for Learning to Fight with Viking Sword and Centre Gripped Round Shield.

BEGINNERS GUIDE – LEVEL 2

by Colin Richards

VIKING SWORD AND SHIELD FIGHTING
BEGINNERS GUIDE – LEVEL 2

Published in Germany
Arts of Mars Books
Colin Richards
31020 Salzhemmendorf
Tel. +49(0)5153/ 80 32 53
http:// www.ArtsofMarsBooks.com

Copyright 2013 Arts of Mars Books

Author: Colin Richards
Design, Photos: Sandra Richards
Copy Editors: Krista Steichen and Carles Barnitz

ISBN 978-3-9811627-4-5

Printed in United Kingdom of Great Britain

All rights reserved. Except for use in a review by a reviewer who wishes to quote brief passages in connection with a review written for inclusion in a magazine, newspaper, broadcast or upon the World Wide Web, no part of this publication may be reproduced or transmitted in any form, without permission from the publisher in writing.

Neither the author or the publisher assumes any liability for the use or misuse of information contained in this book. All martial arts, including historical can be dangerous and should only be practised under the guidance of a qualified instructor, for personal development and historical study.

CONTENTS

INTRODUCTION
Acknowledgements ... 4
About this Book ... 4
The Team ... 6
Before You Start ... 7

SECTION I – GENERAL
I. 1. Historical Background ... 10
I. 2. The Weapons ... 12
I. 3. Safety Equipment ... 13

SECTION II – STEPPING
II. 1. Footwear ... 14
II. 2. Diagonal Half Steps ... 14
II. 3. Combination Stepping ... 22
II. 4. Combination Stepping ... 26

SECTION III – GUARDS
III. 1. Alternate Guard Positions ... 34
III. 2. New Guard Positions ... 38
III. 3. Roof Parries in the Ox Position ... 42

SECTION IV – USE OF SWORD & SHIELD
IV. 1. The Concept of Inside and Outside Line ... 46
IV. 2. Exchanging the Parry ... 48
IV. 3. Disarming the Weapon ... 52

SECTION V – SINGLE PERSON DRILLS
V. 1. Sword Hand Protection Using the Shield ... 56
V. 2. Varying Strike Angled, ... 62
V. 3. Combination Stepping Using Diagonal Half Steps ... 66
V. 4. Combination Stepping Using Diagonal Full Steps ... 82

SECTION VI – PARTNER DRILLS
VI. 1. Combination Strikes Using Diagonal Stepping ... 90
VI. 2. Disarms ... 100
VI. 3. Exchanging the Parry ... 108

SECTION VII – CONCLUSIONS
VI. 1. Common Errors ... 118
VI. 2. An Exchange of Blows - A Fight ... 122
VI. 3. Conclusions

ACKNOWLEDGEMENTS

I must thank my long time friend and confidant Chris Halewood who gave me the inspiration to begin writing this series. Thanks to all the people that have helped, taught and inspired me in the past, too numerous to name.

We must not forget that this book's other two stars are Melvin Raabe and Felix Seidel who stood there patiently for each photo to be taken, even though I had lost my notes of what was coming next. Without them this book could not have been finished. They are always enthusiastic and full of good ideas. Thanks also to everyone else who has contributed to our knowledge and our ideas.

My wonderful wife Sandra Richards and my two sons Jason and Ewan, have inspired me to continue with this work. Sandra has also created the whole design and layout and, furthermore, shot all the photographs.

Colin Richards, Melvin Raabe, Felix Seidel and Sandra Richards hope everyone will find this book useful, and we welcome comments and questions.

All errors that are found in this book are mine and mine alone!

Colin Richards
Salzhemmendorf, Germany
December 2013

ABOUT THIS BOOK

This book contains the second volume of the Viking Sword and Shield Beginners Guides and as such packed with new and interesting theory, drills and exercises. The complete series is designed to facilitate the student in learning to fight relatively safely with the Early Medieval centre gripped large round shield used primarily with a single handed Early Medieval sword or long sax (single edged sword), though any single handed sword could be used.

This Book Series Supports Several Approaches to Combat Simulation
The principles found in this book can be applied to martial arts, stage fighting and re-enactment combat with only a little modification of the techniques and the approach to targeting. Also by applying these self same principles you can adapt the techniques shown to use single handed axe and shield, the short sax and shield and also the single handed spear and shield. Although all of these weapons have technically different handling, most uses of the shield, combat movement, aspects of the thrusting and cutting technique, are identical. We will be addressing the differences between these and other weapons in the next series of books, which will eventually cover all aspects of Viking era combat.

Historical European Martial Art
As a martial art, if sufficient protection is used then you can fight using a full person target, that is all areas of the body can be targeted and hit. Obviously even when a complete and sturdy armour is worn, the dangerous nature of striking the head and throat is reduced, care should still be taken when striking these and other delicate areas.

The main principle of any sword art is control, so that after you have trained enough, you can do anything with the sword, in fact at that level of proficiency your control should be such that no one becomes injured regardless of the type of sword used. Not all of us can become so good, though we should develop enough control so that injury is kept to the absolute minimum. The prime aim of this series is fighting with control. This is because a sword master has absolute control over his weapons at all times, so that he can hit the target aimed for, change an attack into a defence as required or control the extent that a thrust or cut is allowed to travel.

Stage Fighting

When targeting in stage fighting it is usual to target off to the side of the opponent or in certain controlled and practised moves, touching the body. This can be all achieved by slight modification of the targeting principles laid down in these books. Unfortunately targeting off has its own disadvantages as regards safety, and you should not rely solely on that technique. The more able you are to control your weapons the more safe the whole enterprise will be.

Re-enactment Combat

This art is concerned with control and hitting the opponent. The areas that are usually targeted are shown in the first book of the series, though a full body target can be used as well. Of prime importance is controlling the strike and this is achieved through diligent practice and the use of the natural resting position, as detailed in our first book. While taking part in this activity some people do not wear any protection at all, and even though bruising is common, real injury is seldom seen, because everyone trains to keep injury to a minimum.

Fitness and Self Discipline

Of course you can use these books as an interesting and different way of keeping fit and also development of the mind. All the drills and exercises can be combined into a curriculum for increasing your concentration and body coordination, and you will learn a martial art along side even if you never yourself fight anyone.

Training in martial arts should also be fun and engaging, so that the practitioner always feels good afterwards.

ABOUT THIS BOOK

THE TEAM

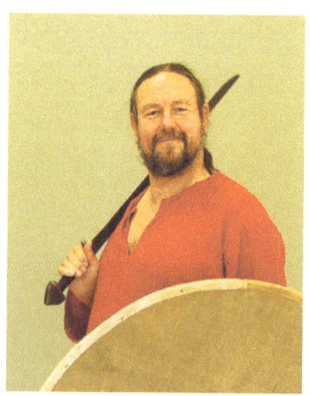

Colin Richards

Born in Liverpool, England, Colin has been interested in weapons, warfare and military history for as long as he can remember. His first steps in martial arts took place 35 years ago when he studied Aikido and various other Asian martial arts.

His main interest lies with the following treatises and areas of research: Viking and Anglo-Saxon Sword and Shield combat AD 400 to AD 1100. The treatises of the fifteenth century Italian Master at Arms, Fiore dei Liberi, this includes many weapon systems. Also the treatise titled in the Royal Armouries Library as 1.33. This manuscript is from around AD 1300 (the oldest of the western European martial arts treatises yet found. Includes: Sword and Buckler combat (small shield).

Colin has taught well over 3000 people in re-enactment fighting and historical martial arts. Having created the Arts of Mars Historical Martial Arts Academy in 2005, he now has over 60 regular students in 4 permanent schools in the Hannover area of Germany.

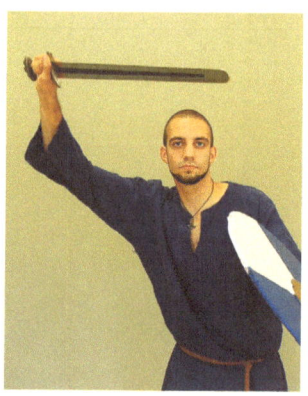

Melvin Raabe

He has been a student of Colin Richards at the Arts of Mars Academy for 4 years. He is training to be an instructor at the academy and learnt to fight with several weapon systems including German Longsword, Sword and Shield, Sword and Buckler, Dusack and Fiore Dei Liberi Dagger. Melvin specialises in German Longsword. He studies Geography at the University of Hannover.

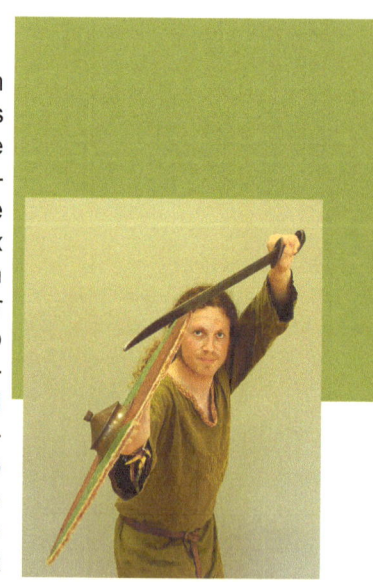

Felix Seidel

Felix Seidel and Melvin Raabe joined the Arts of Mars Academy at the same time and therefore studied the same weapon systems. Felix Seidel specialises in Sword and Shield or Buckler, though he also studies German Longsword, Dusack and Fiore Dei Liberi Dagger. He is training to be an instructor at the academy as well. He studies Geography at the University of Hannover.

THINGS TO KNOW BEFORE YOU START

We wish to promote interest in Historical European fighting techniques. This is the combat heritage of the European people and deserves to be researched and revitalised. People may wish to use this information to study Historical European Martial Arts or for Re-enactment combat, or even for more realistic and historically relevant film and stage combat.

The first book used five attacks and five defences to keep things simple. Each book has added complexity with more guard positions, more attacks and different defences in a way to make learning easier and more fun. In this book the student will find an analyse of how to recognise inside and outside lines, exchange weapons in the bind and disarms a and much more.

This series is called beginners guide, though once you have mastered the techniques therein you will be easily able to fight against people who have vastly more experience though only a poor understanding of the principles used in the fight. This is because they are usually self taught or are taught wrongly by people who have developed tricks which they have made to work for themselves.

Whatever reason you study this weapon combination, of prime importance in every case is control of the weapon and shield. The method of control is described and shown in book one and we advise that every student learns this method perfectly so that the chance to make mistakes in actual simulated fighting as regards to safety is reduced.

How to Use this Book

This book is organised in a simple manner. Each section starts with a few notes that apply to every position in that section, often to the whole book! These notes are followed by pictures which follow in Time Sequence, from left to right. Most pictures have relevant text either above or underneath.

Each picture sits on the Time Line, which is a green stripe which is situated normally two thirds of the way down the page.

Read the Text, drills have a short description of what to do at the start of the drill, position yourself as near as you can to the example given in the pictures and then copy the movements as best you can. After three or four views you should have the basic position and movements in your head. Repeat as many time as you need to.

In some places you will see a close up picture above the main line, this should be used to view the action better. However it may or not be in the correct position relative to the main time line, depending upon space.

If notes are highlighted in red then these are summaries for that section.

The fighter in Red, usually but not always, makes the successful techniques if the fighter in Blue is in the picture. The fighter in Green always shows the technique from the left handed persons perspective.

Grid Lines in the Pictures
Most pictures show a sequence of grid lines on the floor. These are there as a visual aid so that you can better see the distance and angles of steps. We have positioned the lines so that on the left side, when looking at the grid system from the side view, the distance from the first line to the second is a half step, the second to the third a full step, on the right hand side however this is reversed, full step followed by half. The third to the fourth is the weapon range to target. Note we do not always stick to these guide lines as our aim is visual clarity for the reader.

Companion Video
Arts of Mars will be releasing a companion DVD to go with this series of books. This DVD will incorporate all the drills from the three volumes and the theory sections. This DVD will be ideal for you to look at the techniques in full movement. First watch the video and see the moves are put together and then go to the practise session using the book as a reminder.

Companions in Arms
The culture that surrounds any form of recreational fighting with weapons is wonderful. When you fight with someone you develop a special type of friendship and a powerful respect for those you fight and train with. You both know that you are capable of seriously hurting the other person, so that you have to modify the force of your blows and also your intention. Only after you have entered the world of historical armed combat will you realise this for yourself.

We wish you a extremely pleasant and safe experience using the system on offer in this series of books.

BEFORE YOU START

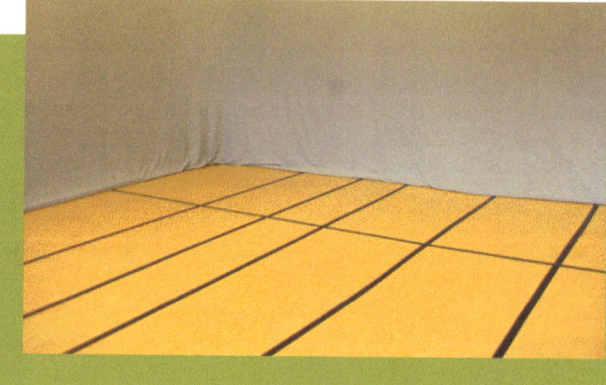

Organisation of the book
We have split this book into four parts. The first is the Introduction, which details useful information, so that the navigation of the material is easy.

Each part is broken down into sections, each dealing with a different aspect, so if the type of information changes so does the section. In the single person and partner drills parts each drill is given a number sequentially so that you can note down the number and find that drill again.

The second is Theory. This is where the actual material is introduced which the book will cover. This is split into easy to identify sections which form logical steps in a learning process, and is essentially the students curriculum.

Thirdly we have Single Person Drills, whereby someone who has either no training partner or they wish to train alone for any reason can do exercises to improve skill levels. These drills as presented in the book are only examples of what is possible. If you wish to get better faster then you must modify the drills to explore other aspects of the example shown. Quite often we provide a few suggestions to help you on your way. The most obvious is to always try starting techniques from different guard positions. Try larger steps or smaller, and also change the angles of stepping and see how that affects the positions. If we are honest with ourselves each book is on average about a years work to perfect the skills presented, so if you have all three books it should take you three years to develop the skills necessary to perform all the drills and exercises from all positions depending on your dedication.

Finally we have the Partner Drills section. This is devoted to developing motion with a partner, so that you can learn correct distance and how that distance changes with angles, and of course timing. These aspects are extremely important in combat, and cannot be emphasised enough. Again the selection of drills shown is only a small proportion of the whole. The student themselves must experiment by making modifications to each drill, ie. start from a different guard, move to a different position and try with another timing.

Please note that this book is written in British English!

BEFORE YOU START

SECTION 1 – GENERAL
HISTORICAL BACKGROUND

Di Grassi
As we noted before virtually the only information about central gripped large shields in a European historical combat treatise that we have found is in Di Grasse's treatise of 1594 in Italian and of 1597 in English. His large shield is different in that it is a rectangle held with one corner uppermost.

He tells us how to hold the big shield. It should not be held against the body even though it would cover all the targets from the shoulder to the thigh. If you wish to rest you can bring in your arm and rest your shield edge on the thigh of the shield side leg.

You must "behold your enemy from the head to the feet" when you hold your shield. This is the first advantage of holding your shield out from the body in the correct position. As we noted in the first book Di Grassi thought that defending against cuts was so easy that he was not going to cover that topic in his book, and would only discuss thrusts. Our research has shown that one of the easiest ways to defeat the defensive potential of a large shield is to convert a cut into a thrust as it nears the shield, so confirming Di Grassi's advise on the subject.

Di Grassi in the second part of his treatise points out that the large shield can defend so easily with small movements that it is possible to open up part of the body as an invitation to the opponent. In regards to smaller shields such as bucklers, he notes that doing this is much more dangerous. This type of tactic is called an invitation. All partner drills in this series should start with an invitation so that the attacker has a target to hit.

The Tower Fechtbuch 1.33
We have also incorporated some techniques taken from the oldest known combat treatise found in Europe, the celebrated 1.33 Tower Fechtbuch.

This book describes a system of sword and buckler fighting which is very sophisticated though not overly complicated. The concept of exchanging weapons such as the shield for a sword in the bind is shown in the 1.33 treatise and is known as the Schildschlach, or shield hit. This is used to control both the opponent's sword and shield at the same time, so as to release their own sword for an attack. Though re-enactment fighters had discovered how

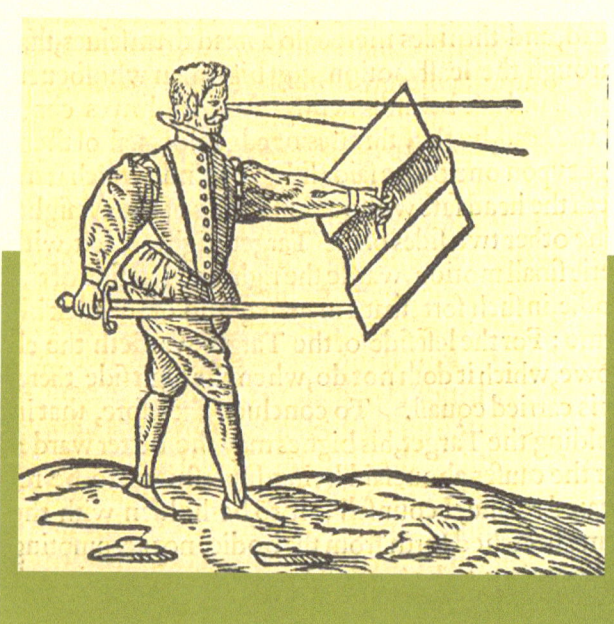

This is a picture of his large Target showing how it is held and where to look.

to exchange weapons before 1.33 was discovered by the HEMA community, nevertheless the principle used is the same.

Also most of the guard positions we use are from the 1.33 treatise, though some we have taken from the German Longsword tradition.

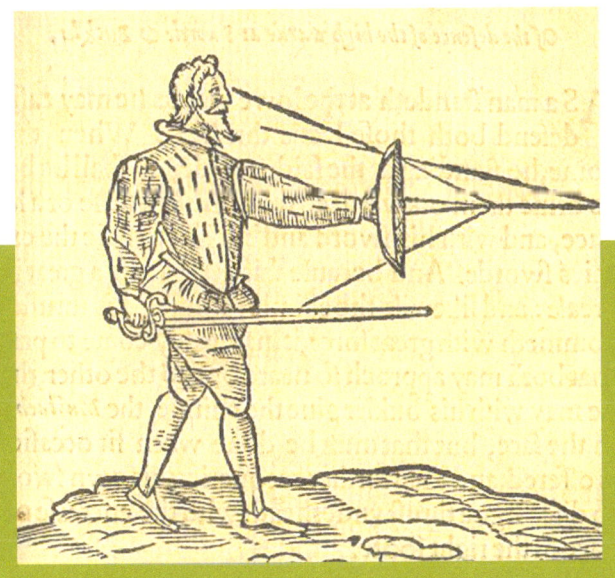

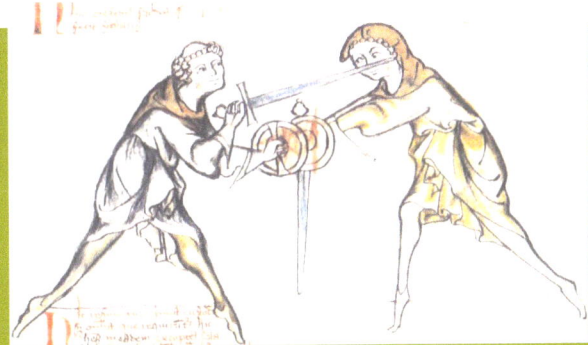

This drawing is from Di Grassi's book showing how and where the buckler is held in his system

This an example of a schildschlack or shield hit, used to control the opponent's weapons, releasing the sword to be used to attack.

THE WEAPONS

The Sword
In books two and three we have swapped to using sprung steel weapons because this is the normal weapon used for re-enactment and martial art combat in Europe. We recommend training with nylon or plastic weapons to save the metal weapons for actual combats. We will give various web addresses at the end of the book where you can obtain such weapons.

The Shield
We have used for the most part a smaller shield than normal, with a diameter of about 24 inch or 60 cm **in order to be able to see the techniques easier.** We have also used a shield with a diameter of 85 cm to show that the technique used **can be influenced by the size of the shields themselves.** We have tried to stay faithful to the technical sequence regardless of the size of shield. Where you find difficulty using your own shield in a particular technique sequence please modify the technique used to suit your type of shield. You will also note that in some pictures the attacker or defender has no shield. This is again to **facilitate the students view of what is taking place,** in the proper situation both people would be armed accordingly.

Note that Viking era shields seemed to have varied in diameter between 60cm and 90cm, with some even larger possible. The greater the diameter of the shield the more difficult it is to do several things from the attackers point of view.

Firstly manoeuvring your own sword around your shield becomes more problematic the larger it is. Essentially the variation in the type of attack is reduced, because of the physical interference caused by the shield.

Secondly the amount of target exposed on the opponent is less, therefore limiting the type of attack that will cause a displacement of the opponent's shield. Which means it will be hard to get the opponent to expose an area long enough to hit it!

There are other disadvantages also, not least, the weight will tire the opponent much quicker, making stamina an important factor in the fight. There are other traits of large shields that we will look at in the Advanced guides, and we will look at further ways to defeat large shields in that series of books.

The Concave Shield
We present an alternative shield design, the concave shield. This is depicted in various books and paintings and so enthusiasts have built them to see how they handle. We do not recommend that someone new to this type of combat uses them as you must develop slightly different skills to be effective. We will discuss these shields in later volumes.

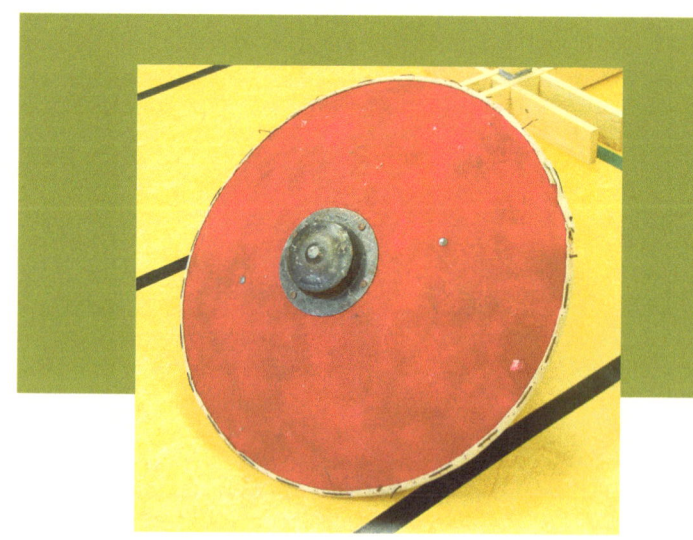

SECTION 1. 2.

SAFETY EQUIPMENT

We highly recommend the use of protective equipment whenever you take part in combat. This should protect delicate areas and especially the head, throat, groin and hands. See the Beginners Guide Book 1 for further details.

Pell
The pell is identical to that shown in the first book except we have added two more tapes in green. The uppermost indicates the arm pit or upper arm of the target. The lower level with the stomach or even upper thigh. This is so that we can demonstrate that blows from above and below can be redirected to lower or higher targets. All tapes are positioned to the height of the person who is using the pell relative to their body.

Recommendations
We recommend that you practice these drills with substitute weapons to save the blades of expensive steel weapons. Practice weapons are made from a variety of materials including wood, plastic, nylon, padded carbon fibre rod, and bamboo covered with leather. If you would like to see more information about these weapons and steel swords please look at our web site www.Swordexperts.com.

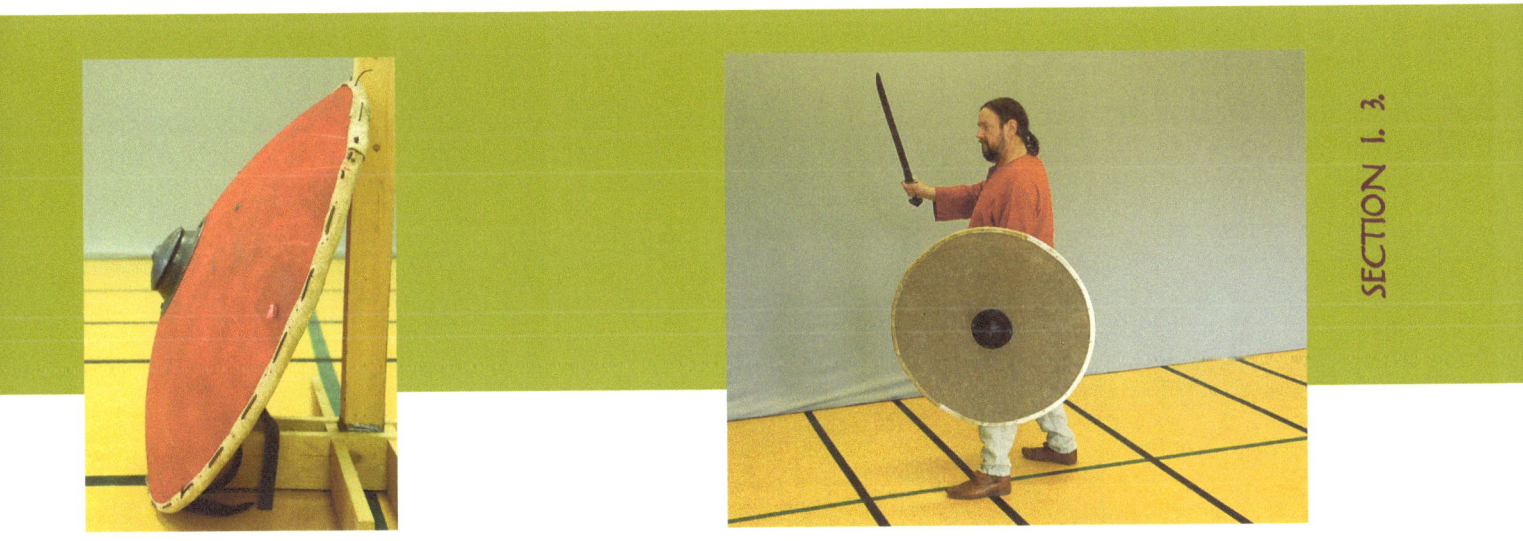

SECTION 1. 3.

SECTION II - STEPPING

FOOTWEAR

We have covered some of the more common steps in the first volume, such as forward and diagonal full and straight half steps going forward.

How you move and where you move is very important and will determine how the fight plays out, especially if you are fighting against multiple opponents. Footwear also influences how you move. Modern training shoes and similar footwear give several advantages and also disadvantages compared to the historical turnshoe of the Viking Era. The modern shoe allows a more secure movement on wet or slippy terrain, the rubber sole giving a better grip. They are also better at protecting the feet from injury on a wider selection of ground conditions than the turnshoe. On the other hand turnshoes allow you to feel the ground better as they are thin and flexible, which can be a great advantage in certain conditions, such as ground with holes or protruding objects in the surface. They are also better at allowing the foot to turn quickly in almost any terrain.

Weight Position
We recommend that you still keep your weight evenly distributed over both legs, until you are comfortable with stepping and striking in all directions. A fighter must also be able to negotiate all types of terrain while fighting and so you should practice your footwork in different ground conditions. Try in wet grass, stone floors and woodland, you will quickly appreciate the different footwork needed. In wet conditions it is best to keep the width of stance small and in woodland while engaged in fighting you have to feel with your feet as you move.

DIAGONAL HALF STEPS

Exercises 1-4
We now examine half steps done at an angle going forward. For convenience we show these made at approximately 45 degrees, though you can vary the angle as required due to the situation.

These are very useful for varying position in a fight, and when combined with other steps can greatly increase the tactical possibilities. Firstly we will look at half steps going left, starting with the left leg for-

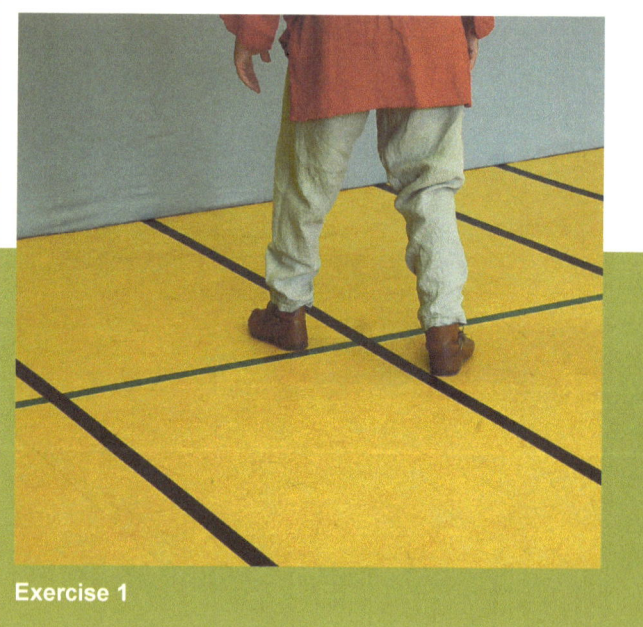

Exercise 1

Left leg forward. Weight in the middle in normal stance.

ward, and then with the right leg forward. These steps are excellent for keeping the shielded side to the opponent while moving round their unshielded side. When fighting the left handed person this manoeuvre is typical for both combatants as they both wish to protect the unshielded side and also threaten the opponent's unshielded side by moving to that side. In a shield wall this usually leads to the end man, if left handed, either turning inwards on the line and collapsing it or drifting off to the left. Exactly the same happens in the other battle line if the last man is a right hander. It requires experience to prevent this from happening.

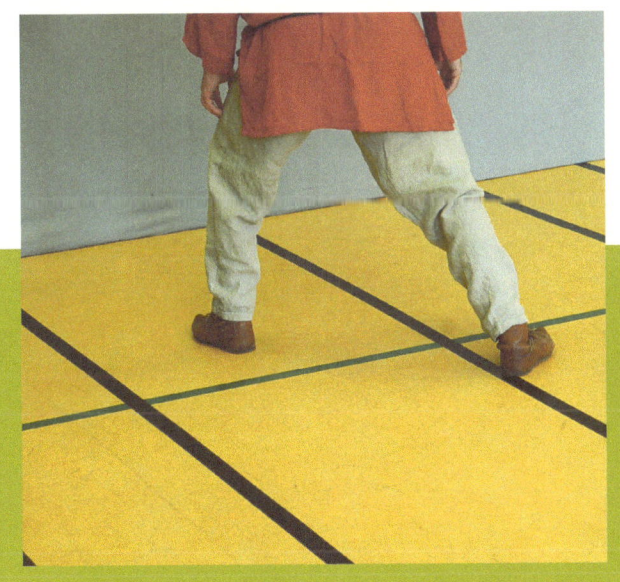

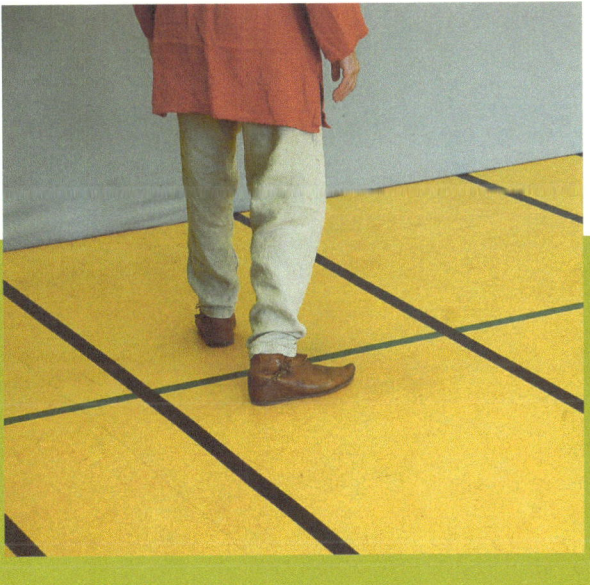

Make a half step approximately 45 degrees from straight ahead to the left.

The back foot moves up to re-establish the original stance.

In this case the right leg is forward, though the step is to the left. This manoeuvre is used to engage the opponent's weapon side with your weapon, see later the section on exchanging parries for some uses.

If the opponent seeks to retreat slightly then the angle of the step could be reduced to around 20 degrees to the straight ahead, sometimes this is enough to offside the opponent's defence. The opponent should seek in response to either re-establish the central position or move off the new centre line created by the movement of the other player. This movement and counter movement is the essence of combat and is best exploited by good timing, and accurate footwork.

Remember the greater the angle of step to the side of straight ahead, the shorter the forward movement. This means that offline movement shortens the fighter's reach relative to the opponent's initial position. This can be critical as the opponent only has to slip a little back to become out of reach against off line steps. This can be done very quickly.

Through experience the angle and length of step become an automatic choice, as does the follow on technique.

SECTION II. 2.

Exercise 2

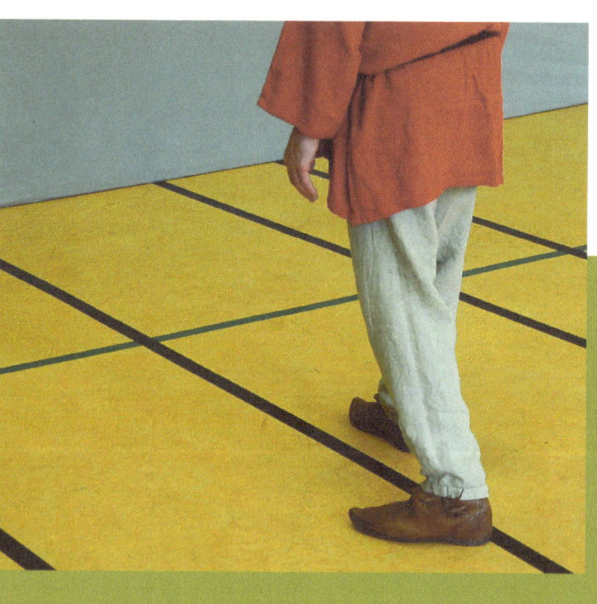

Right leg forward. Weight in the middle in normal stance.

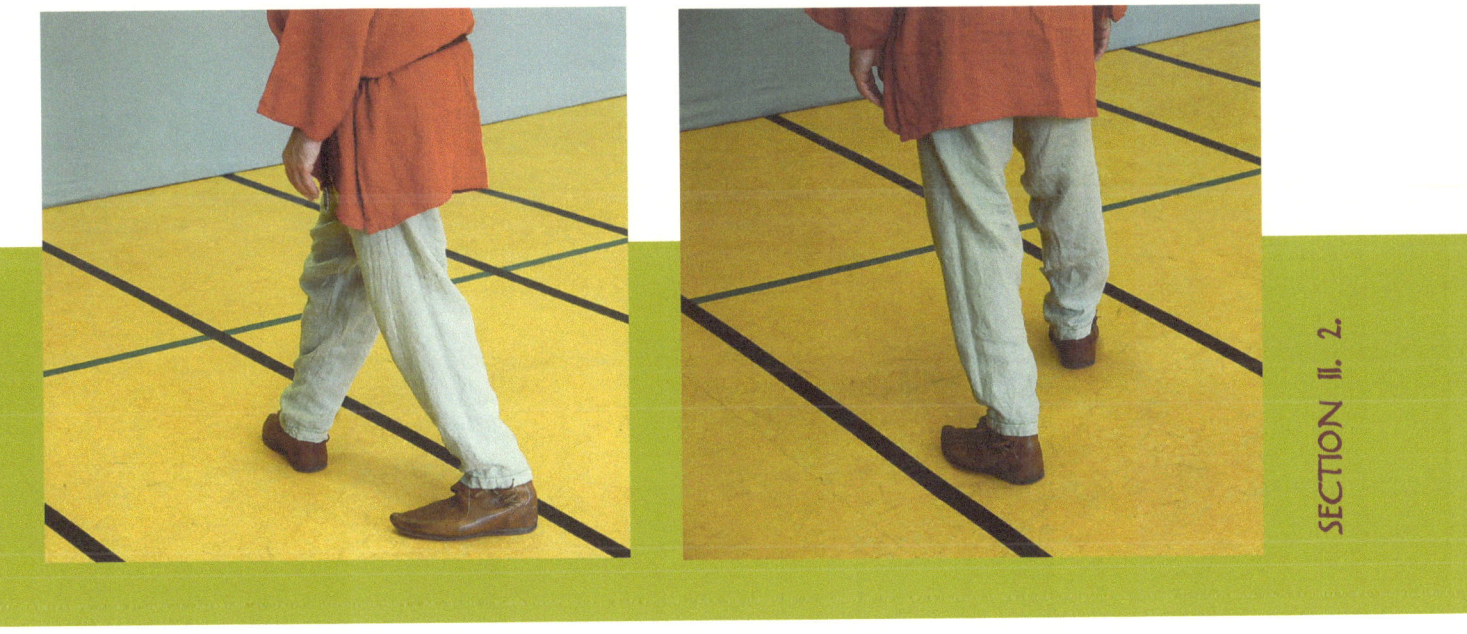

Make a half step approximately 45 degrees from straight ahead to the left.

The back foot moves up to re-establish the original stance. Notice the body has turned to the right slightly to orientate the body to the target and therefore the power.

SECTION II. 2.

Now the half steps will go to the right. The first has the left leg forward, and is one of its uses is to slip further away from the opponent's weapon side, while simultaneously bringing your weapon closer. The added benefit is that the shielded side is presented to the opponent.

This is the typical movement of the right handed person against a similar sided opponent, even though the other fighter is presenting his shield and seems well protected, there is a real benefit moving away from the opponent's weapon. The defender must adjust position immediately or be in danger of being beaten with a quick technique that circumvents the shield.

SECTION II. 2.

Exercise 3

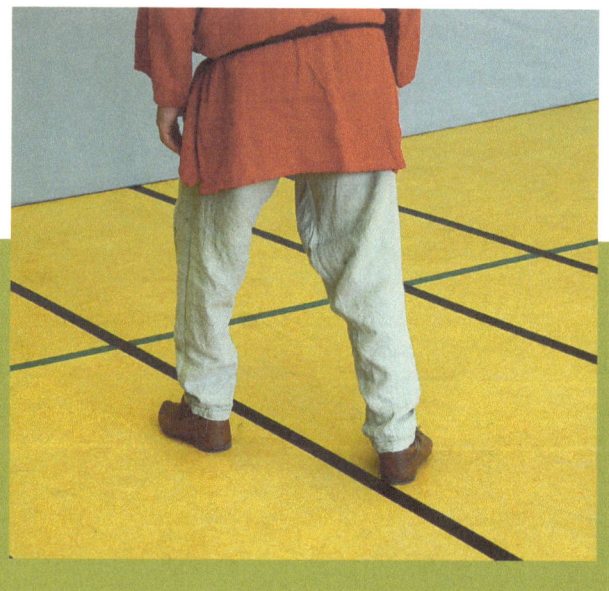

Left leg forward. Weight in the middle in normal stance.

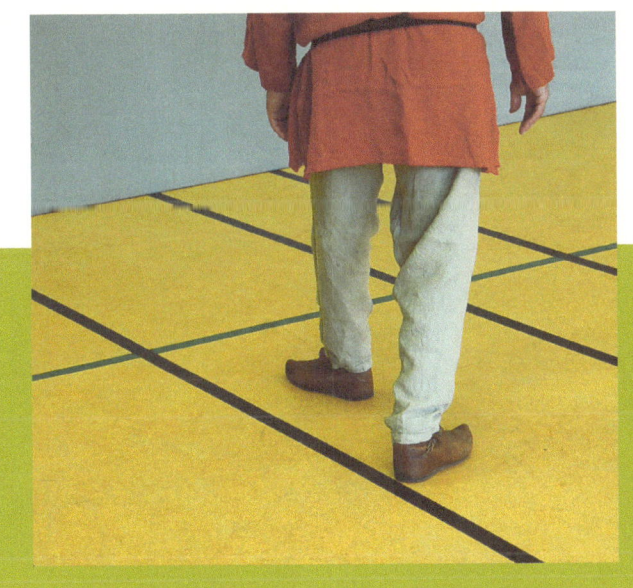 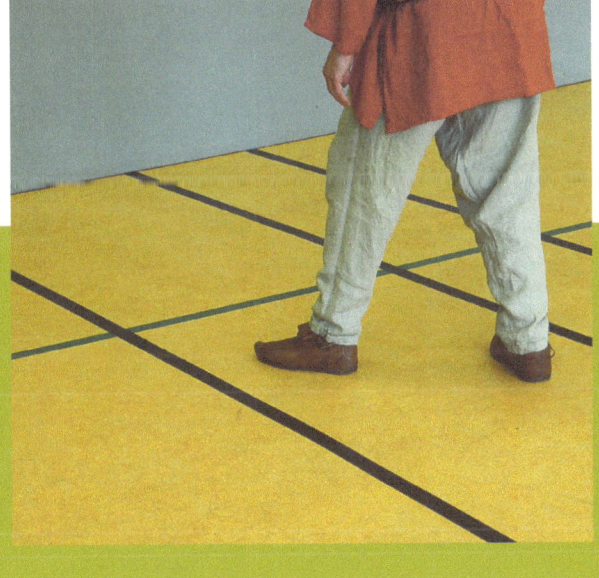

SECTION II. 2.

Make a half step approximately 45 degrees from straight ahead to the right.

The back foot moves up to re-establish the original stance. Notice the body has turned to the left slightly.

This time the right leg is forward and the fighter goes to the right. This has similar advantages to the last movement, though the weapon reach is further enhanced. If the timing is right this step is also excellent at avoiding attacks to the left shoulder, even without a parry.

The fighter can repeat several of these steps in a row to move even further around the opponent's shielded side, changing back to the other side with a diagonal step with the back leg, switching the line of attack quickly to advantage. The opponent has to counter each move or find himself in an awkward position very quickly.

SECTION II. 2.

Exercise 4

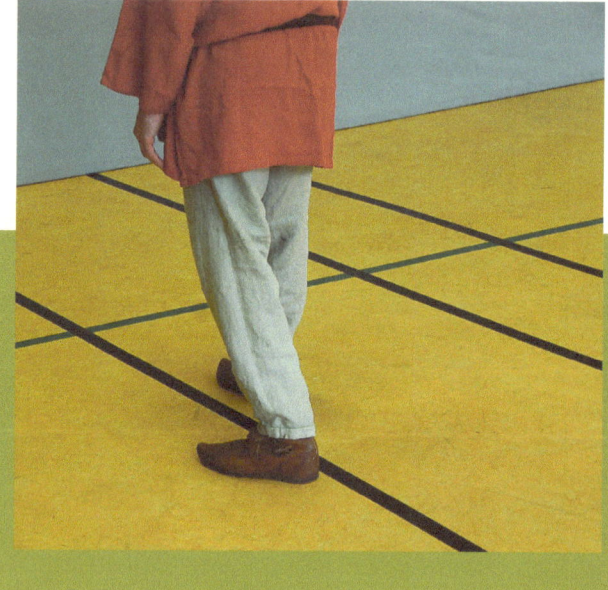

Right leg forward. Weight in the middle in normal stance.

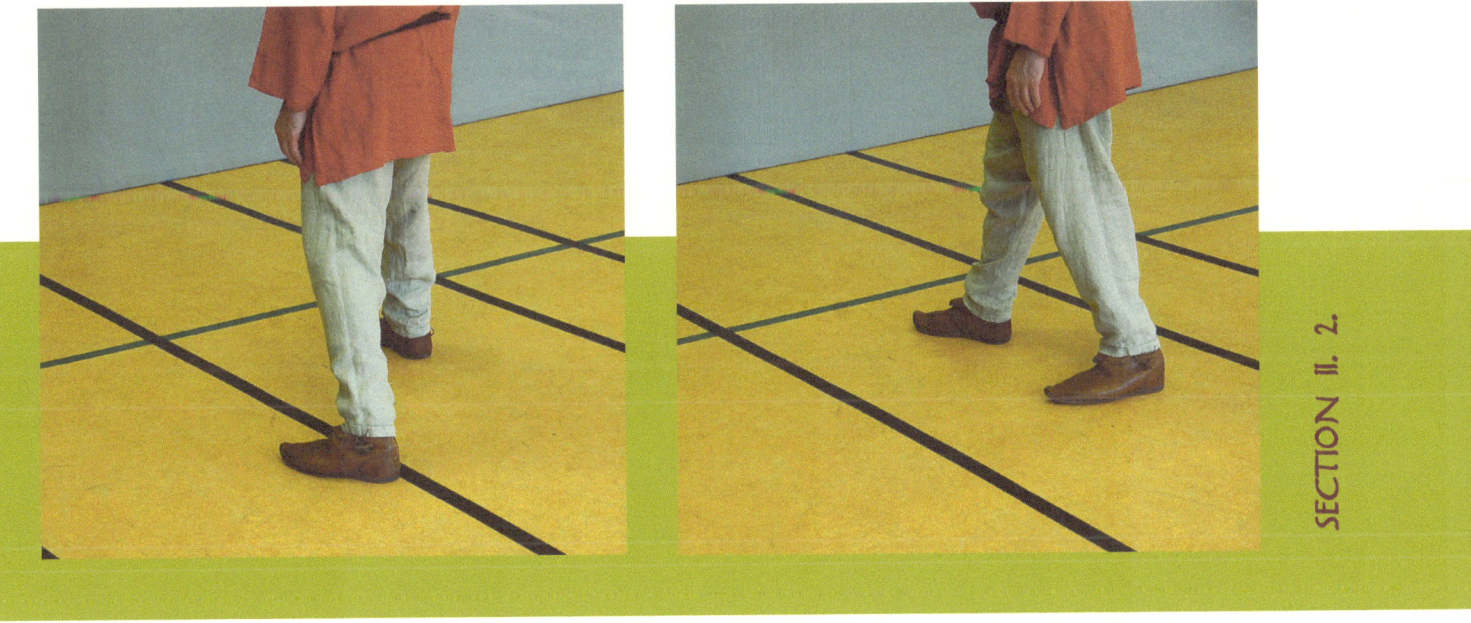

Make a half step approximately 45 degrees from straight ahead to the right.

The back foot moves up to re-establish the original stance. Notice the body has turned to the left slightly.

COMBINATION STEPPING – FIRST METHOD

Exercises 5-6

Half Step, Full Step Combination

In combat, fighters do not make one step and stop. This would end up with very staccato fights and look very strange. Most fighters combine steps into effective tactical sequences in order to try and secure a better position from which to fight from, which is usually from the side or rear.

There are endless footwork combinations that we could analyse, though here we will concern ourselves with only two. These are the half step, full step and the full step, half step manoeuvre which everyone can train to create powerful tools to use in their combats.

We follow a half step forward, with a diagonal full step to the side producing a movement off line to the opponent's centre. In this example this foot-

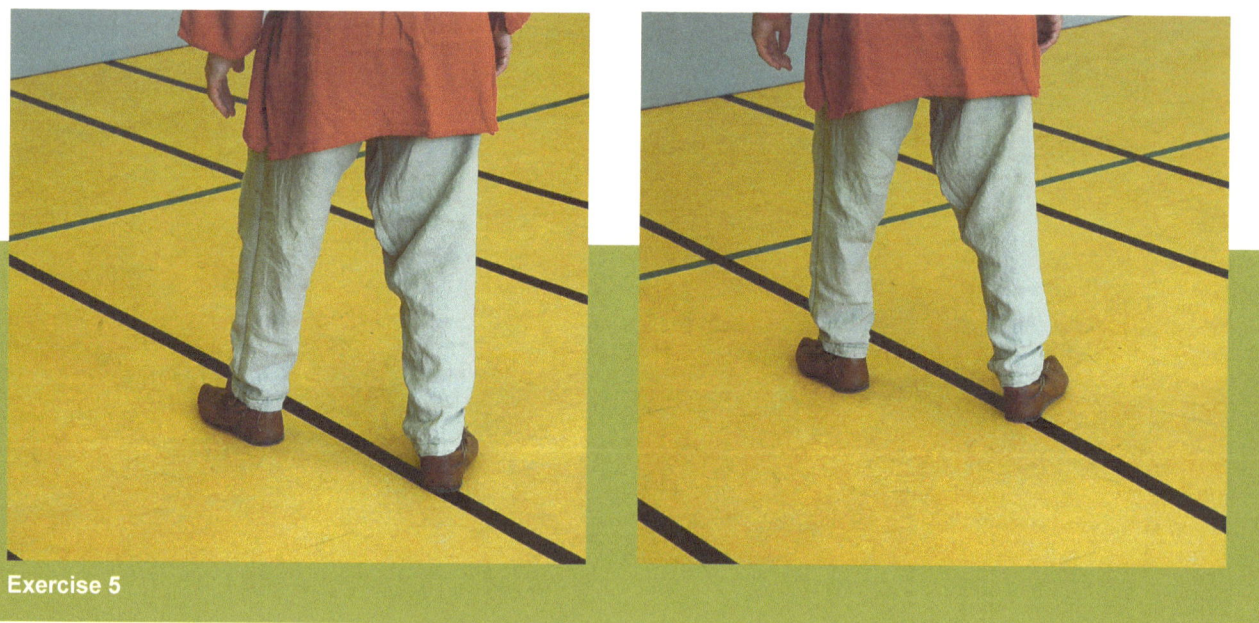

Exercise 5

Start in the normal stance, left leg forward.

The front foot steps directly forward. The back foot moves up to maintain stance.

work is used to move round to the shielded side of the opponent and therefore further away from the opponent's weapon.

This is a very powerful move if the timing is right and combined with a vigorous or even a sneak attack. The aim of the attack is to panic the opponent into freezing in place, so as they cannot attempt a counter movement. Inexperienced opponents often either stand in place or only turn, without maintaining distance, which leaves the completely open to forward diagonal movement and combination strikes.

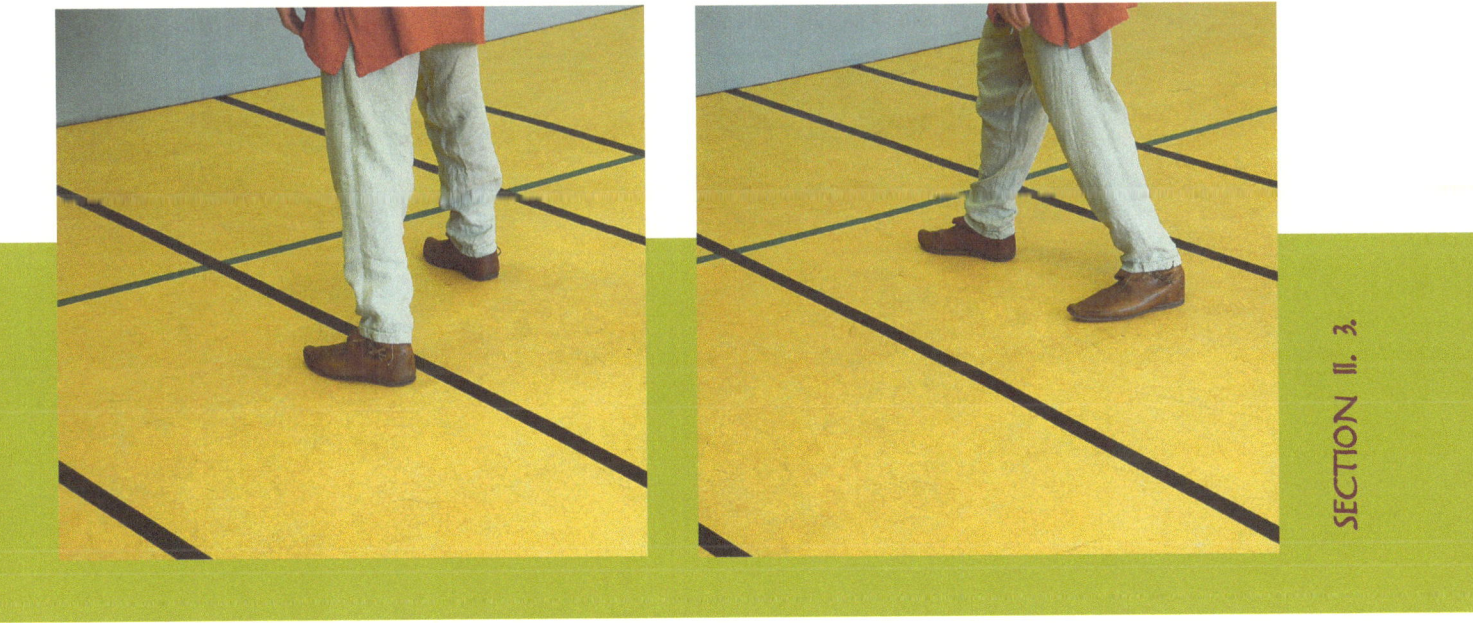

SECTION II. 3.

The back foot steps diagonally to the right at about 45 degrees.

The back foot steps behind the front foot re-establishing normal stance.

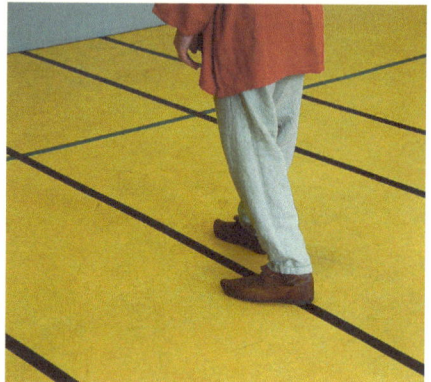

Start in the normal stance, right leg forward.

If the right leg is forward we can use the same footwork to move around to the unshielded side of the opponent. This footwork is very important when we discuss combination strikes and feints [see next level of guides], as it allows you to move to either side of the opponent and forces them to react or be left at a positional disadvantage.

This manoeuvre also helps dominate the opponent's weapon, you have positioned both your sword and shield against his weapon, which means that both can deal with it adding extra security and control if needed.

SECTION II. 3.

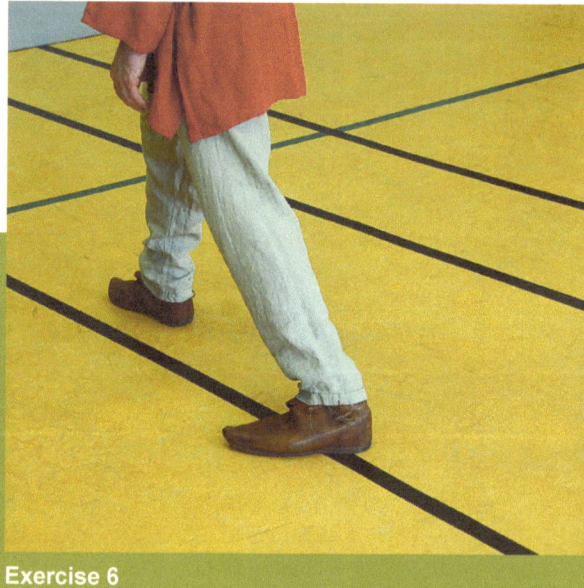

Exercise 6

The right leg steps directly forward.

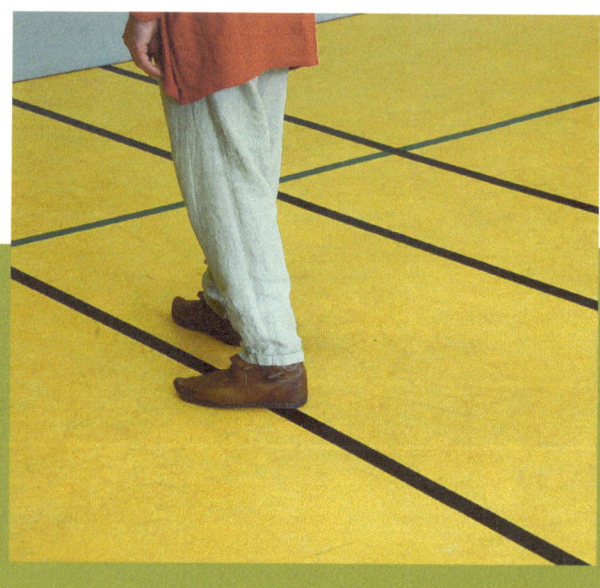

The back foot moves up to maintain stance.

These combinations can also be made going in the other direction as proposed in these examples. So after half stepping forward with the left leg, do the full step diagonally to the left with the right leg. After half stepping with the right leg forward make the full step diagonally to the right with the right leg. Then move the back leg to re-establish the correct stance. These steps are cross steps, that is the rear leg crosses over in front of the leading leg. These steps are inherently more difficult to execute and so we will cover them in far greater detail in the advanced guides as they have many interesting tactical uses. For the moment the fighter should be aware that these steps are possible.

The more options you have in footwork the more chance you have to outwit your opponent in the heat of battle. These simple alternatives mean that you can turn the opponent any which way and keep the initiative, probing for weaknesses and trying new approaches.

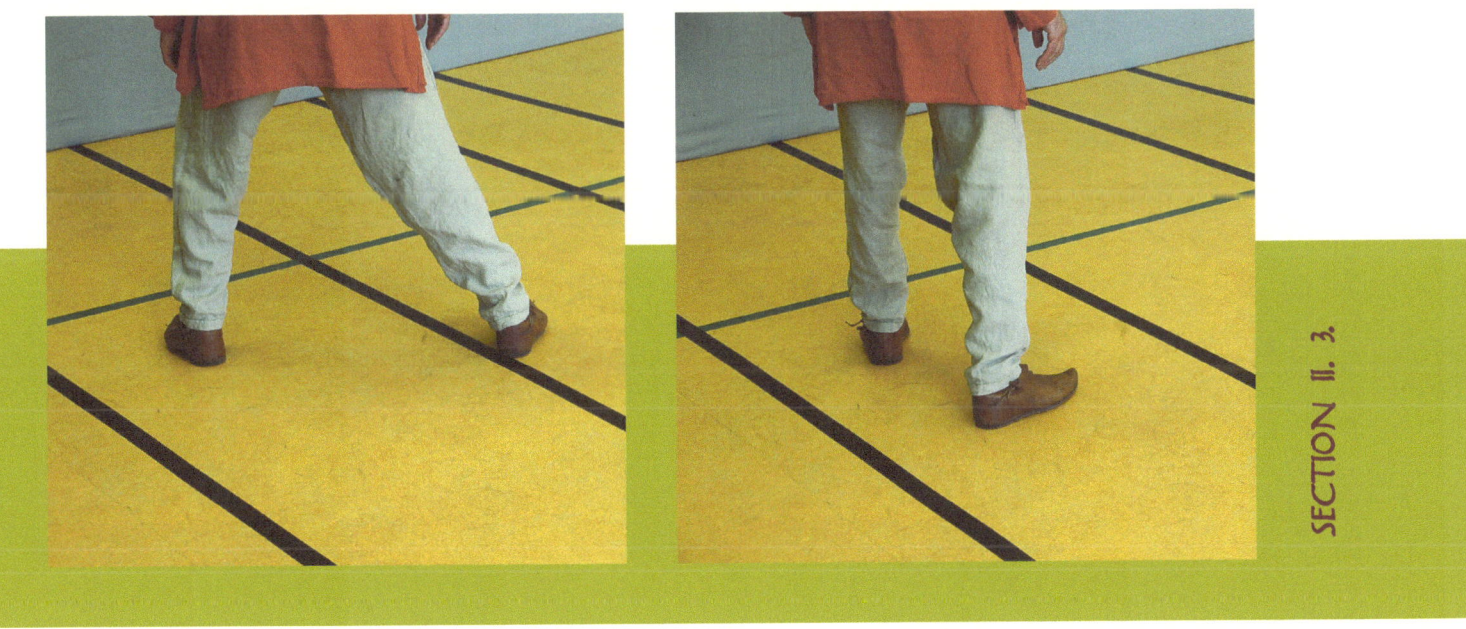

The back foot steps diagonally to the left at about 45 degrees.

The back foot steps behind the front foot re-establishing normal stance.

SECTION II. 3.

COMBINATION STEPPING – SECOND METHOD

Exercises 7-10

Full Step, Diagonal Half Step Combination
We always recommend to engage the opponent at about one and a half steps away, so that there is time to develop a defence against a quick attack, and also to give distance to develop tactics by combining different attacks with different footwork.

These tactical nuances will become more apparent as we progress through the curriculum. Here we show and describe some of the more simple though effective combination steps. In any given step: as the first foot lands going forward, orientate the stance in line to the target. Going backward, orientate the stance in line to the target as the second foot lands.

Left Leg Forward
Here with the left leg forward, the combination starts with a full step forward and then goes to the right using a half step. This closes distance quickly

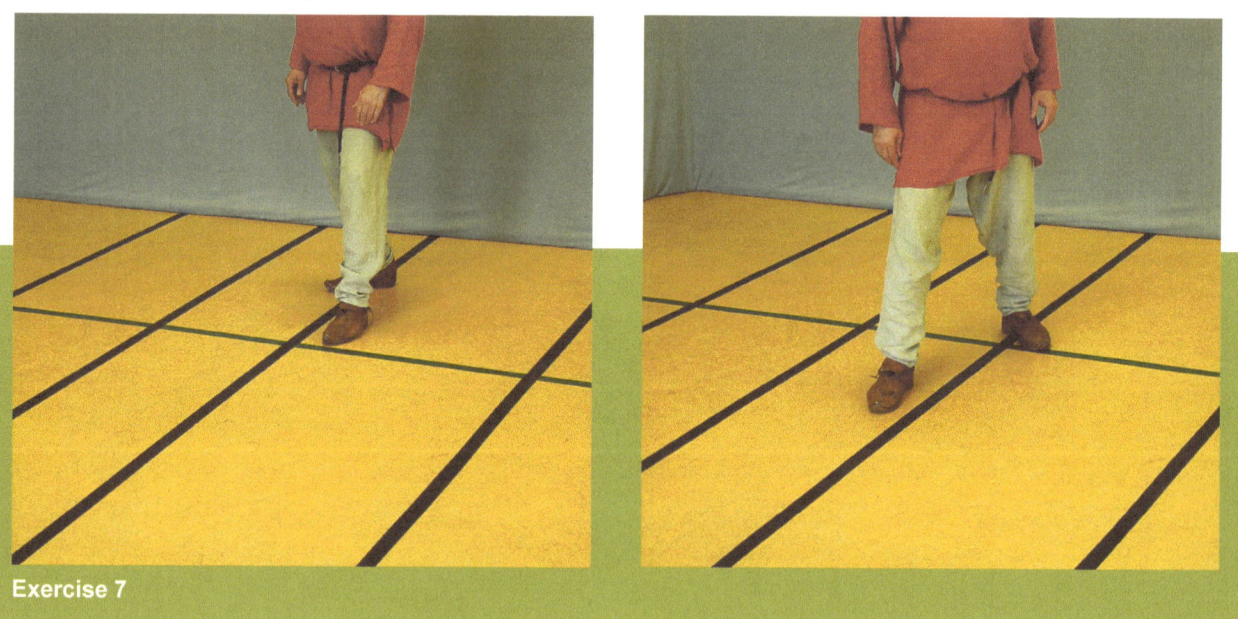

Exercise 7

Full Step, Half Step Combination Going Right
Start in the normal stance, left leg forward.

The right leg steps directly forward.

and moves away from the opponent's weapon side. Swapping to the weapon side forward also increases reach and develops a positional advantage if the opponent does not turn to maintain their centre line on the attacker.

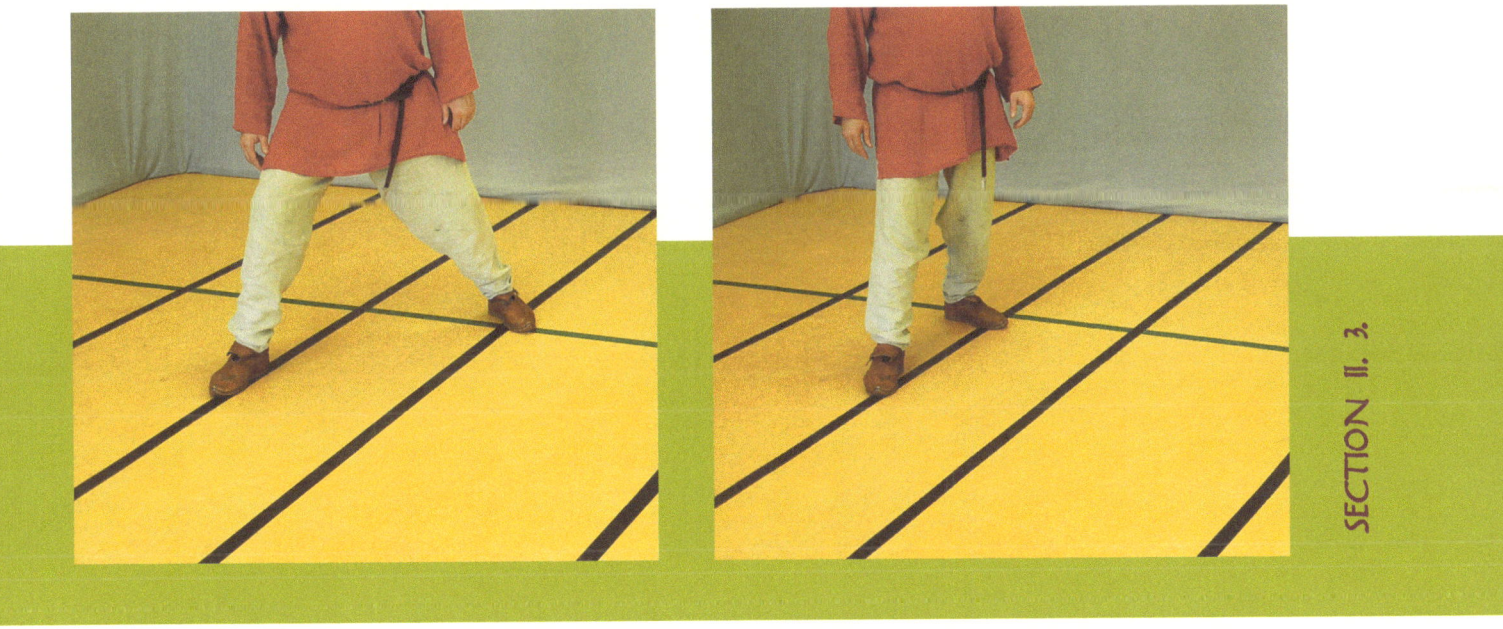

The right leg then steps diagonally to the right at about 45 degrees.

The back foot steps behind the front foot re-establishing normal stance aligned to the opponent.

SECTION II. 3.

Right Leg Forward

If the right leg is forward we can use the same footwork to move around to the unshielded side of the opponent. This footwork is very important when we discuss combination strikes and feints [see next level of guides], as it allows you to move to either side of the opponent and forces them to react or be left at a positional disadvantage.

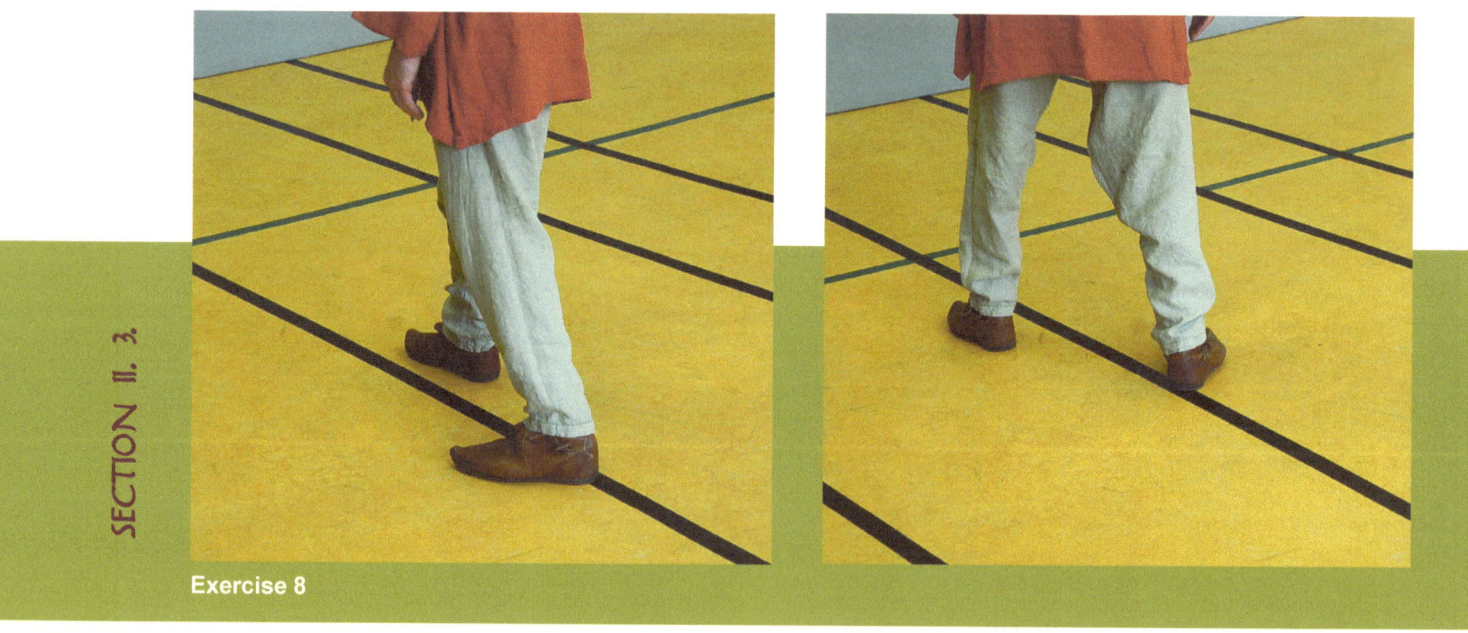

Exercise 8

Full Step, Half Step Combination Going Left
Start in the normal stance, right leg forward.

The front foot steps directly forward. The back foot moves up to maintain stance.

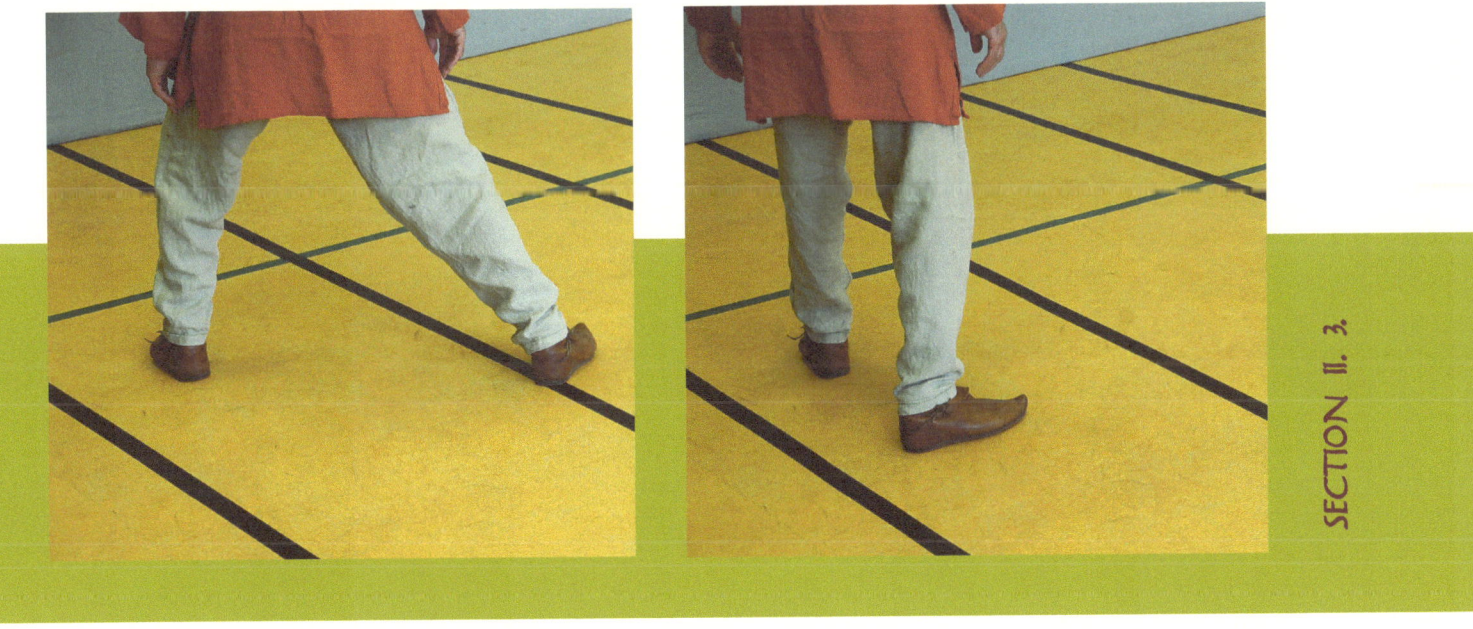

The left leg then half steps diagonally to the left at about 45 degrees.

The back foot steps behind the front foot re-establishing normal stance aligned to the opponent.

Left Leg Forward
Here by moving with the half step to the unshielded side we attempt to close down the opponent's weapon by presenting the shield forward while giving them a positional disadvantage. It takes practice to do these manoeuvres without exposing your own unshielded right hand side as you move.

SECTION II. 3.

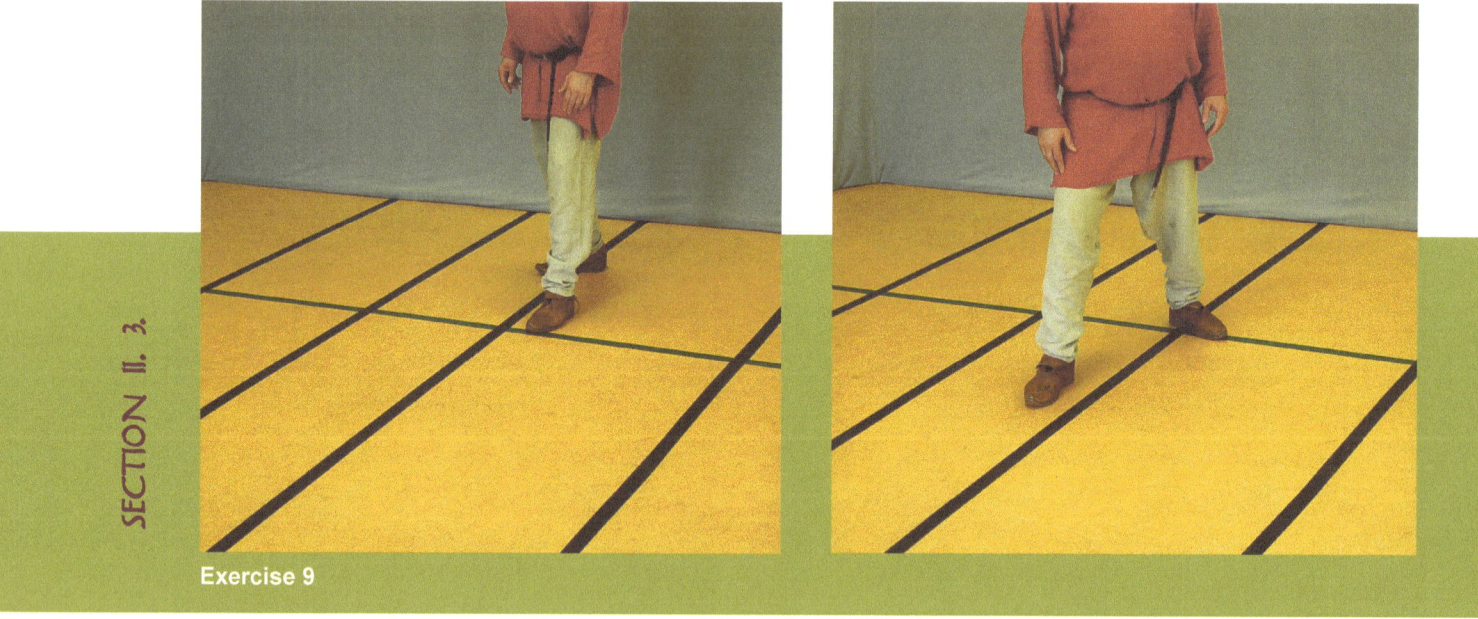

Exercise 9

Full Step, Half step Combination Going Left
Start in the normal stance, left leg forward.

The right leg steps directly forward.

Both this and the next example are actually cross steps, though the cross is done with a half step. This type of cross step is both quicker and easier to execute than the full cross step we mentioned at the end in Combination Stepping Method 1. The end effect is similar to those steps though there are differences. The true cross step where the rear leg moves forward can lead to stability issues during the movement, which can be exploited if the opponent knows how to take advantage of this.

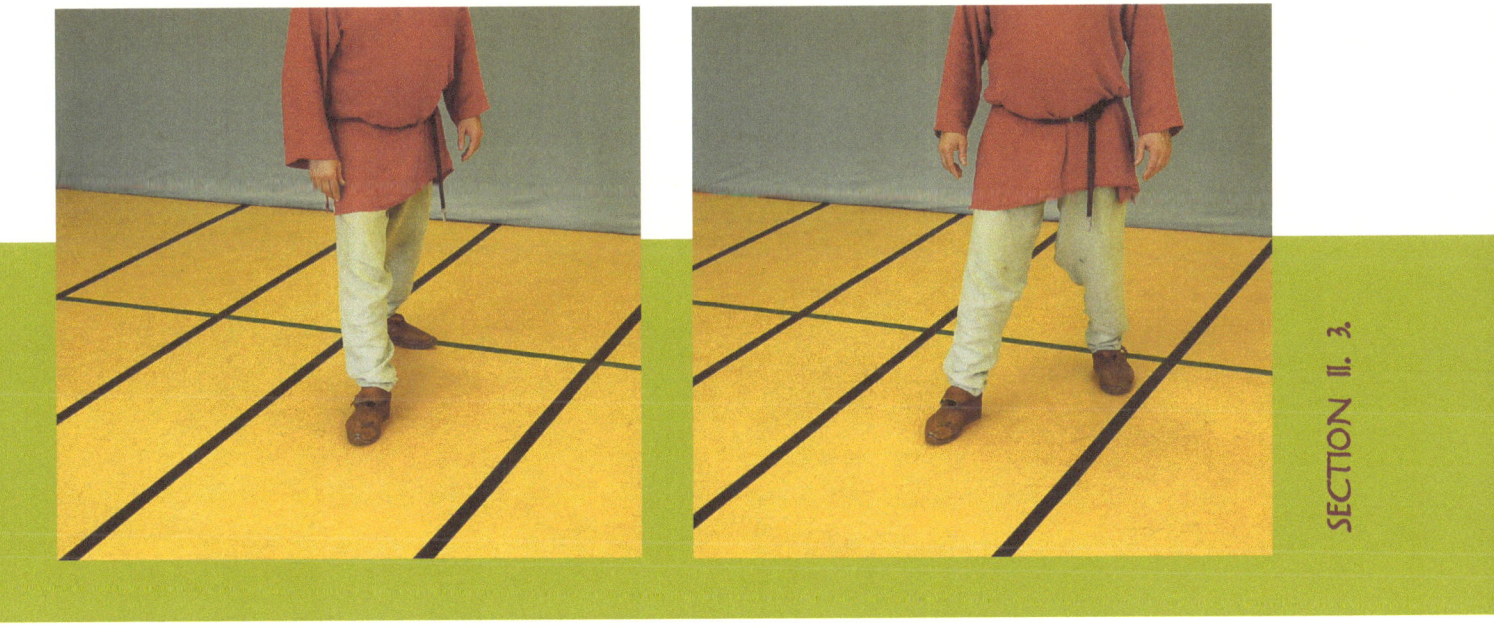

The right leg then half steps diagonally to the left at about 45 degrees.

The back foot steps behind the front foot re-establishing normal stance aligned to the opponent.

Right Leg Forward

The object of this manoeuvre is to move to the opponent's shielded side while keeping the shield side forward, simultaneously moving away from their weapon side.

This maintains full shield security and pressures them tactically, psychologically and physically; this triple threat can cause inexperienced fighters' defence to collapse. Further half steps can be made in this same direction in succession to keep the pressure on the opponent.

On the other hand by simply stepping diagonally with the rear leg further to the right, though at a small angle, can bring the sword behind the shield's defensive line, if the fighter does not react in time.

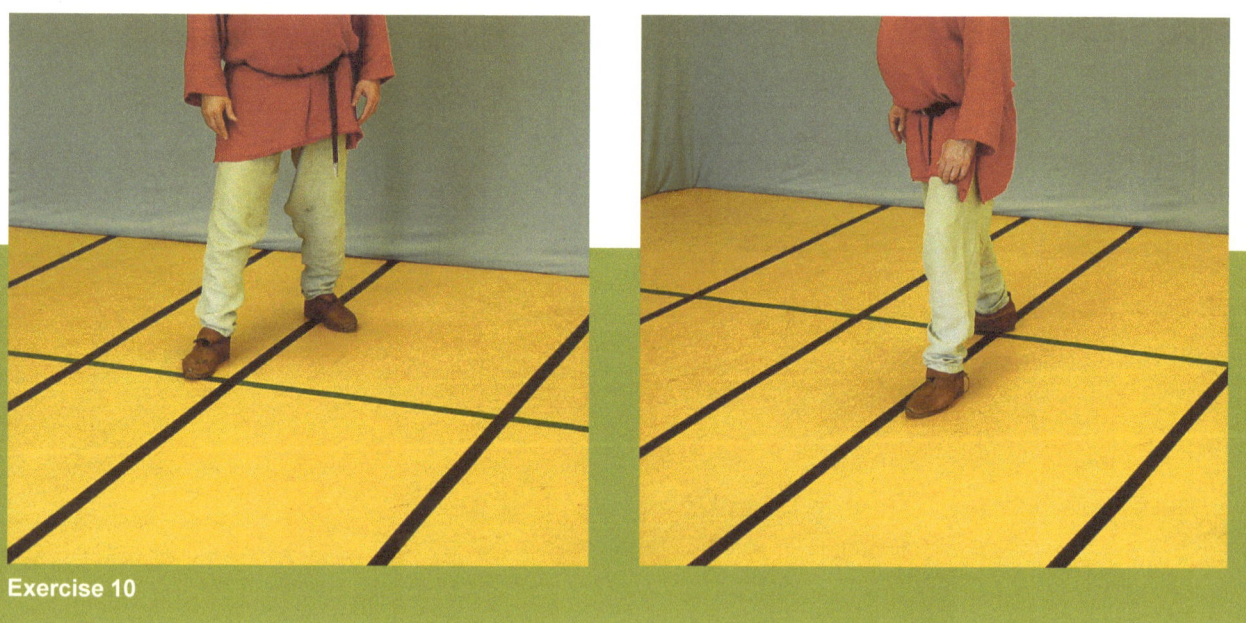

Exercise 10

Full Step, Half step Combination Going Right
Start in the normal stance, right leg forward.

The left leg steps directly forward.

Summary For Stepping

- As the first foot lands going forward, orientate the stance to the target.
- As the second foot lands going backward, orientate the stance to the target.
- Diagonal steps can be of any angle dependent upon the situation.
- Width of step is dependent upon the terrain and the distance you wish to traverse.
- Smaller steps are generally quicker, and half steps quicker than full.
- Stepping too wide can lead to instability.

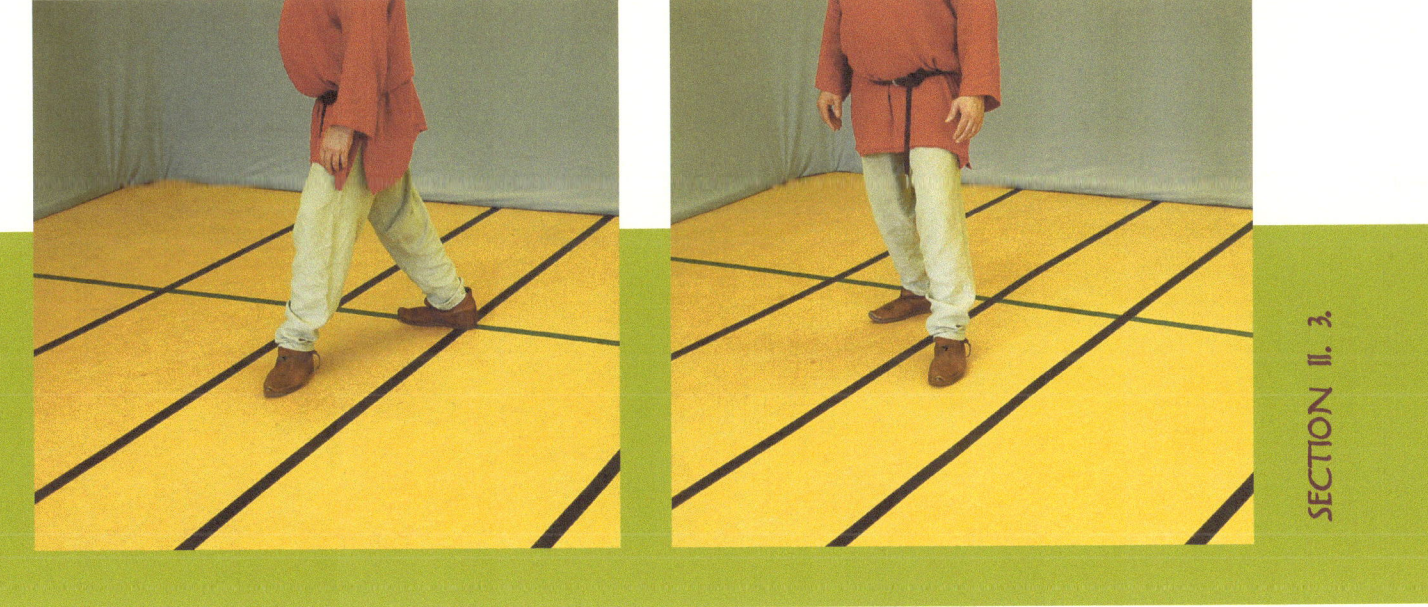

The left leg steps diagonally to the right at about 45 degrees.

The back foot steps behind the front foot re-establishing normal stance aligned to the opponent.

SECTION II. 3.

SECTION III – GUARDS
ALTERNATE GUARD POSITIONS

Purpose and Use, Introduction

In this volume we will develop the number of guard positions to give more flexibility to the fighter's options. Firstly we can slightly modify the ones already studied to give them subtle differences which the fighter can use to his tactical advantage. This usually takes the form of invitations to attack certain areas. For instance a combatant can feign tiredness and lower the shield so that the left shoulder and head is uncovered. Similarly we can alter the position of the sword to lure people to attack the exposed shoulder when actually the fighter can cover that area with the shield, the sword is only waiting to counter attack when the time is right. The student should try and invent their own invitations by modification of the guards, and experiment with ways to lure the opponent into prepared positions.

Guard Position Modifications
Use as Invitations

In this example the shield is held high and the sword is moved into a low position, this is known as in German Longsword terminology as "Fools Guard", because it looks foolish, or maybe because only a fool would attack it without thinking first.

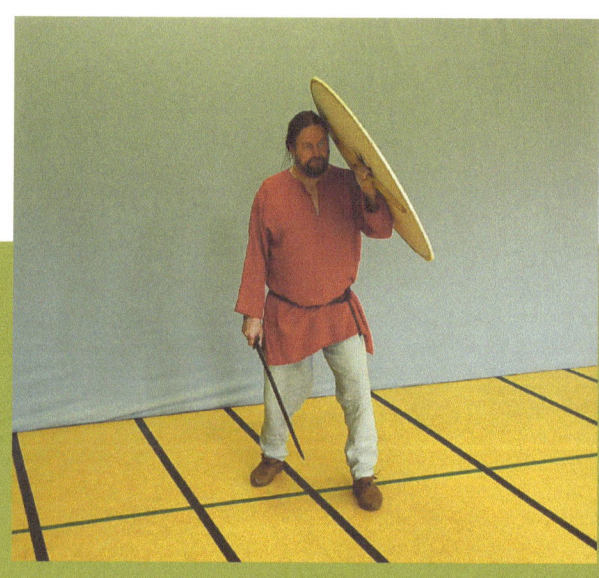

Shield High, Sword Low
The shield covers the high line, the head and shoulder, the sword the low line.

This position also exposes the whole lower left side which is easily defended by a quick movement of the shield or sword. Be sure not to blind yourself with the shield. The upper right side is also exposed.

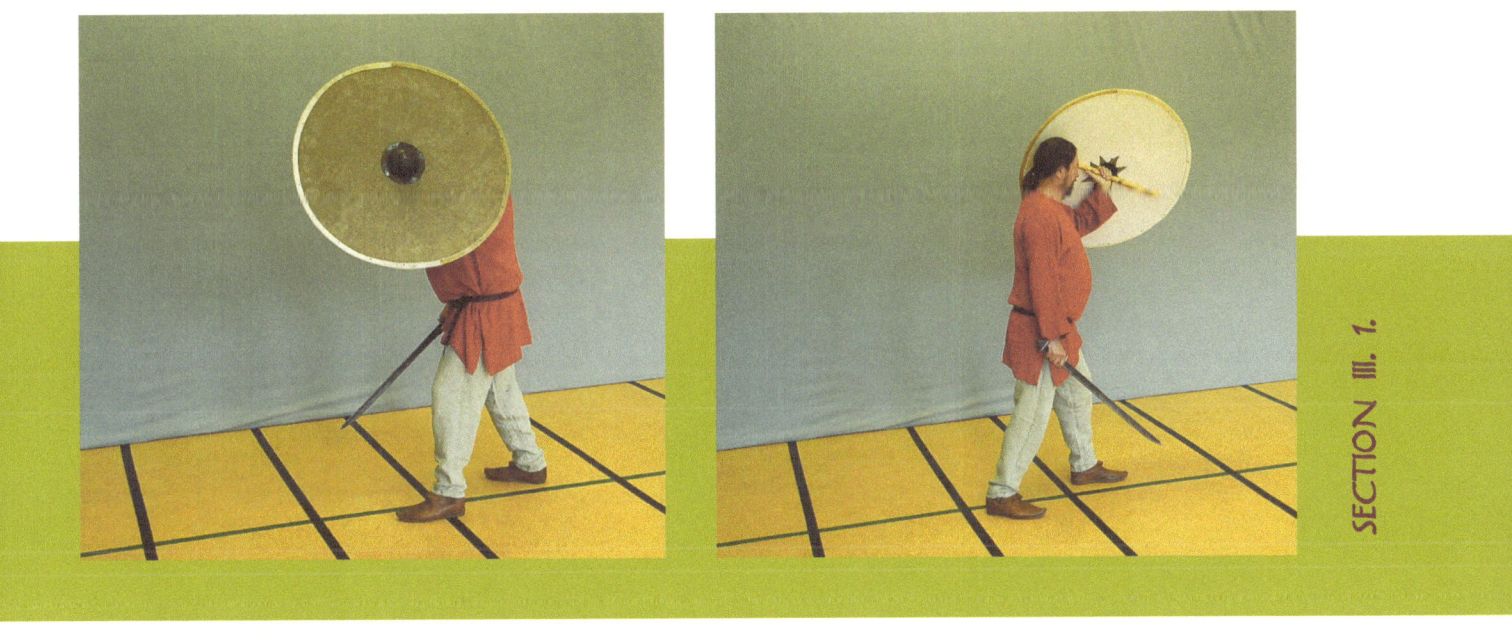

Do not blind yourself with the shield. The sword can parry any attack to the legs.

This position open up the lines to the right shoulder and body.

Here is an invitation to the left shoulder. Used carefully it can lure an opponent into attacking into a prepared defence. Raise the shield to parry as the attack comes in, just one option is to attack the sword arm as it comes in while stepping to the side. See later in book 3.

You can also block with the sword and exchange the parry with the shield, see later in book 2.

SECTION III. 1.

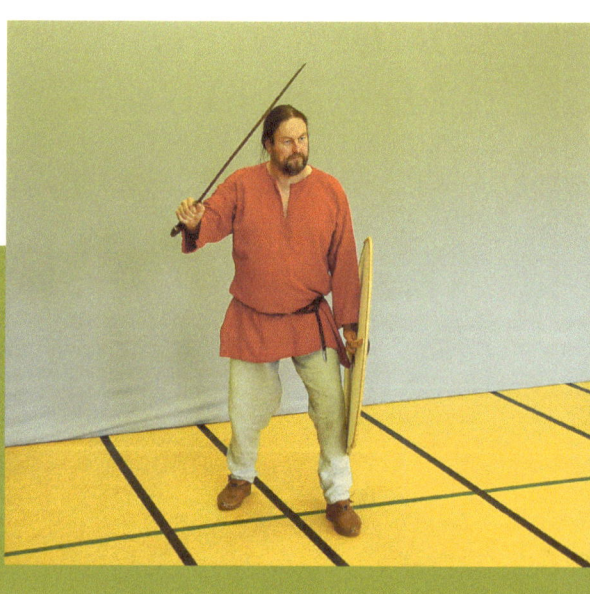

Shield Low, Sword High
The sword covers the high line, the head and right shoulder, the shield the low line.

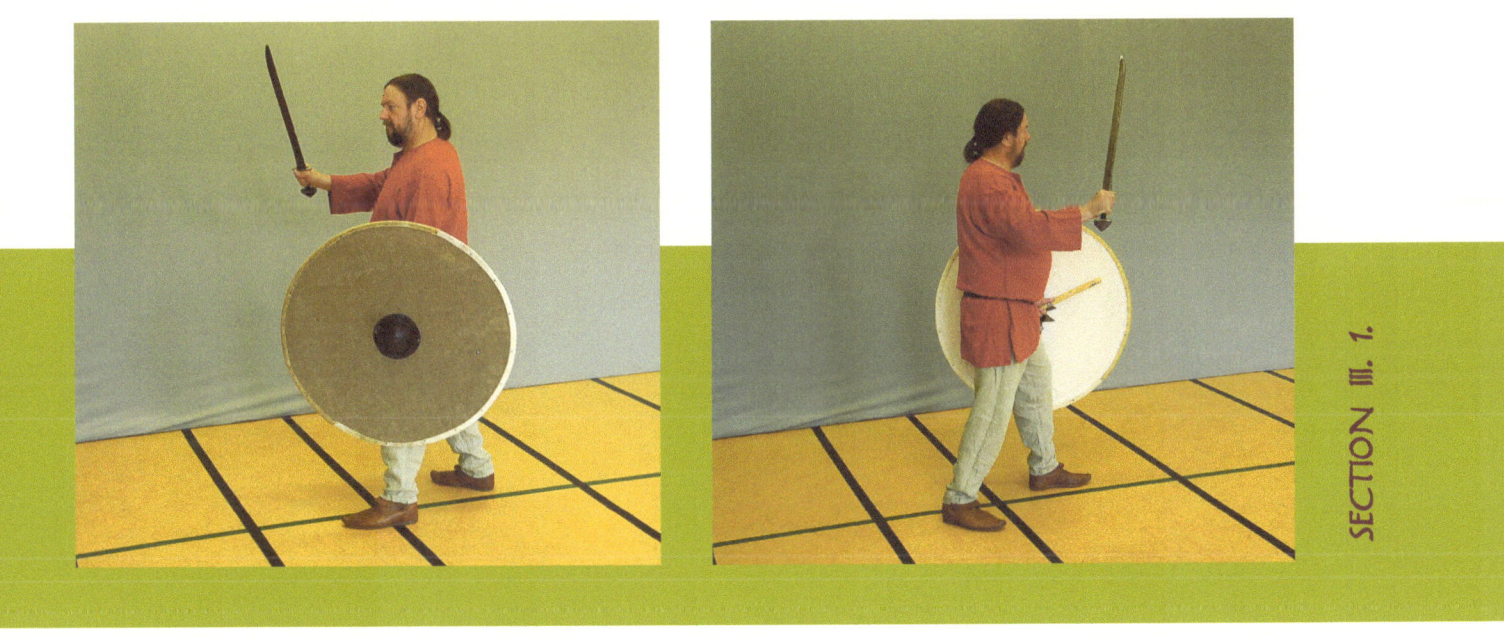

The shield can parry an attack to the shoulder if raised and lower legs if the stance is dropped.

This position opens up the lines to the left shoulder and head.

SECTION III. 1.

NEW GUARD POSITIONS

Ox Guard
This guard is good to stand in as the sword is ideally situated to block attacks to the head and shoulders. It is a standard position in many martial arts, and in German Longsword it is called the Ochs/Ox position, because the position of the sword resembles the horns of the ox when made on either side. This is an excellent name and so this book will recommend that students use it too.

Right Ox
When in the guard position the point of the sword is aligned with the face of the opponent. This naturally guards the right side of the head and the shoulder against diagonal attacks.

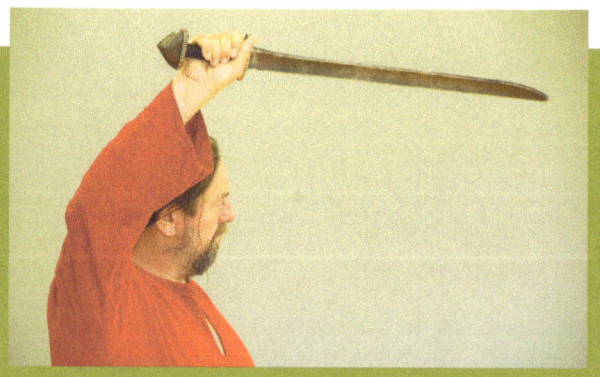

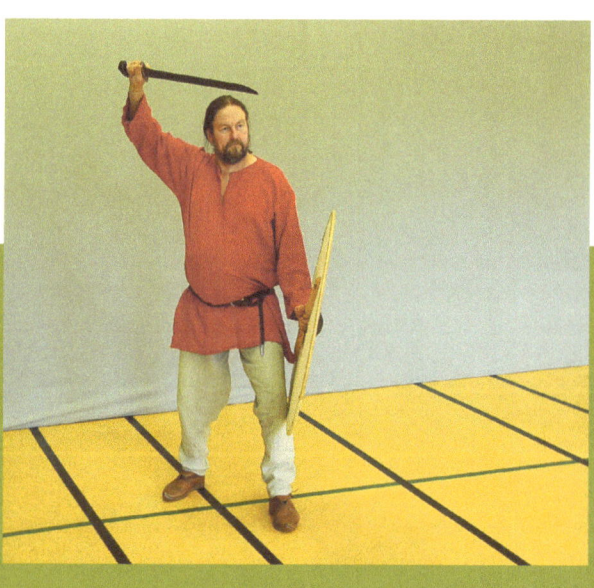

The sword covers the high line, the head and right shoulder.

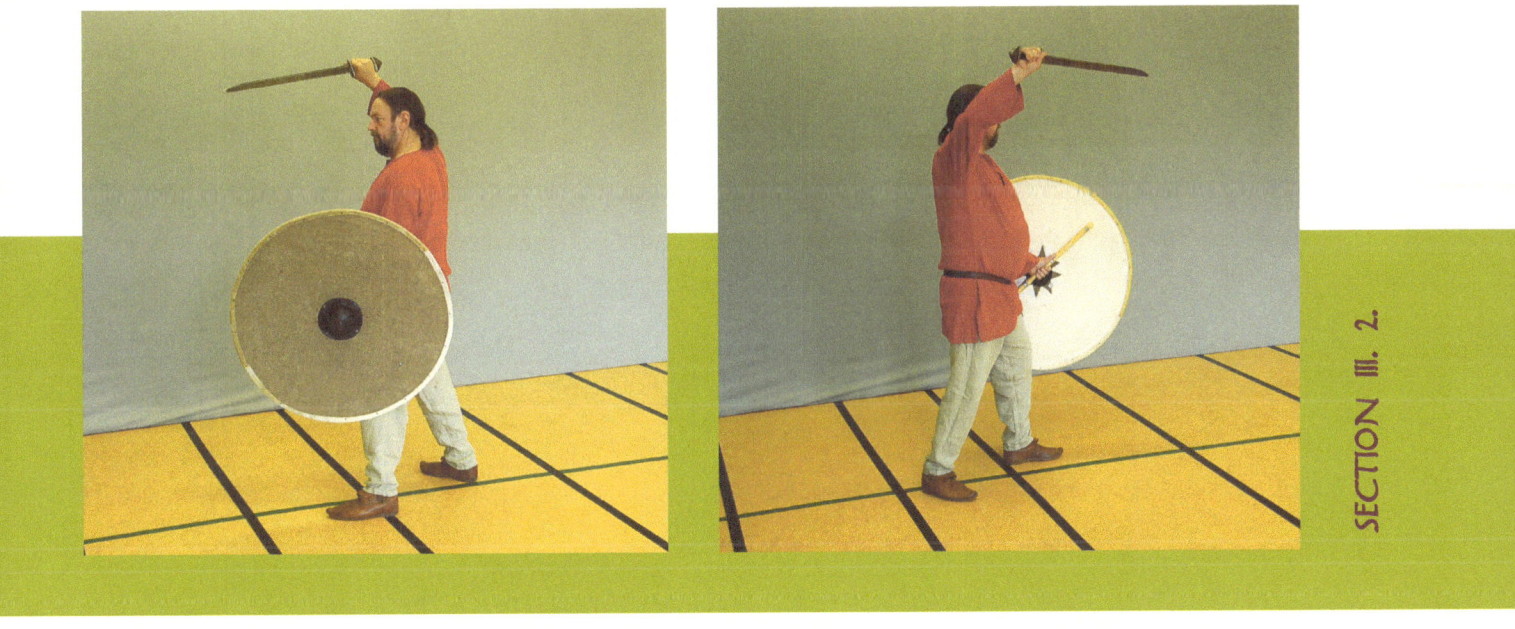

The sword can parry an attack to the right shoulder and head.

Note the position of the blade of the sword is forward and above the head, so that a blow never reaches the head even if the sword is depressed a little.

Left Ox
When in the guard position the point of the sword is aligned with the face of the opponent. This naturally guards the left side of the head and the shoulder against diagonal attacks.

These positions are excellent for all round defence of the upper body, and are easy to attack from, either with a thrust or a cut. The main drawback of these positions is that defending the legs with the sword is more difficult due to the large distance they are from that area. Usually with a large shield that is not a problem. Left ox in particular is slightly awkward at first and exposes a large target area to the opponent, unless they are left handed.

SECTION III. 2.

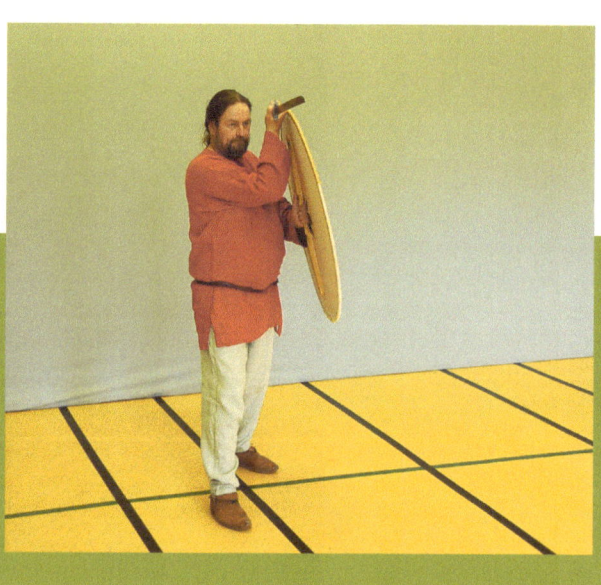

The sword and shield covers the high line, the head and left shoulder.

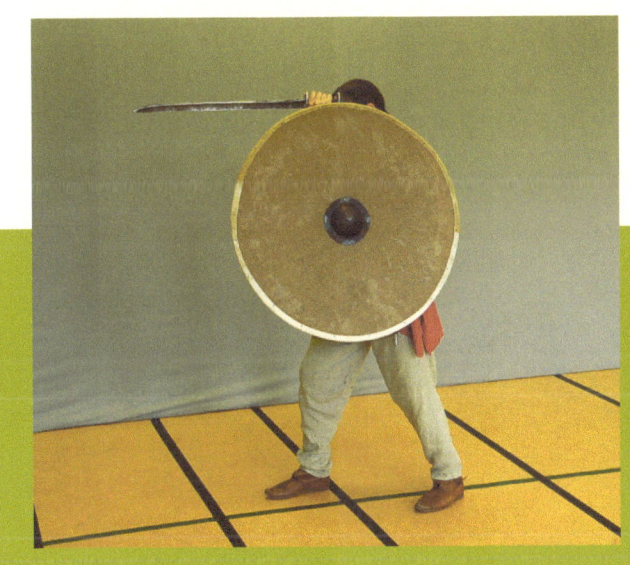 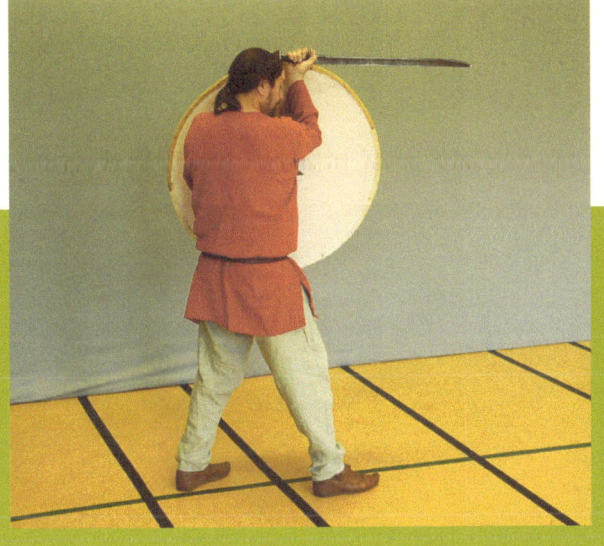

The sword could parry an attack to the left shoulder and head.

Note the position of the blade of the sword is forward of the head, so that a blow never reaches the head even if the sword is depressed a little.

SECTION III. 2.

ROOF PARRIES IN THE OX GUARD POSITION

By simply modifying the position of the sword in both these Ox positions we can use these guards to defend the other side of the head and shoulder. The the sword is simply pointed approximately 45 degrees to the other side and the sword hand is brought nearer the centre and this makes what is commonly known as a Roof Parry.

This is again right Ox position, though with the blade hanging to the left so that it can cover the left shoulder and head.

You can also drop the point even further to cover lower targets, though reaching the lower part of the legs will be difficult to execute quickly due to the distance the sword has to move. See Parry 4 from the first volume.

When parrying the hand is exposed, so that it is important to parry with the point forward and so that the distance is such that the attack cannot hit the hand. Changing the angle of an attack is simple, reacting to pull the hand out of range at the last moment is not.

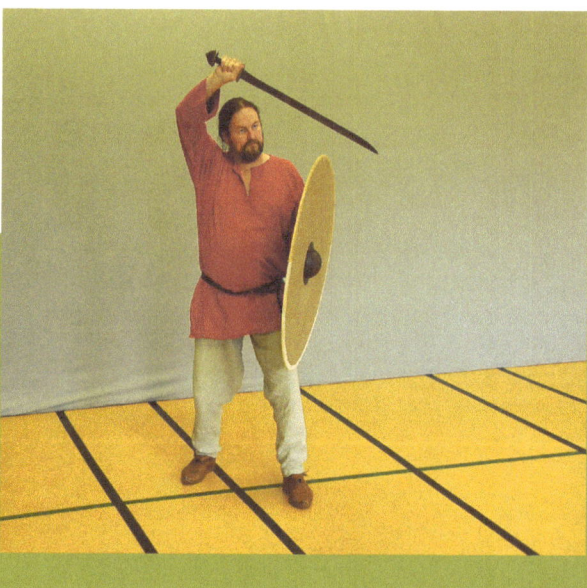

The sword point moves over and covers the high line, the head and left shoulder.

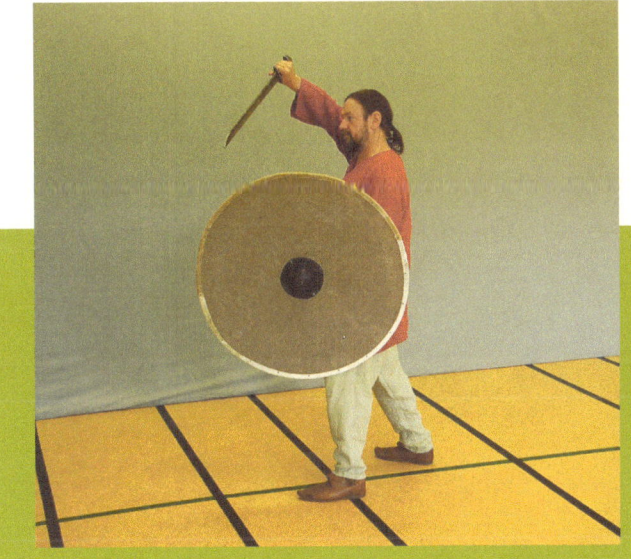 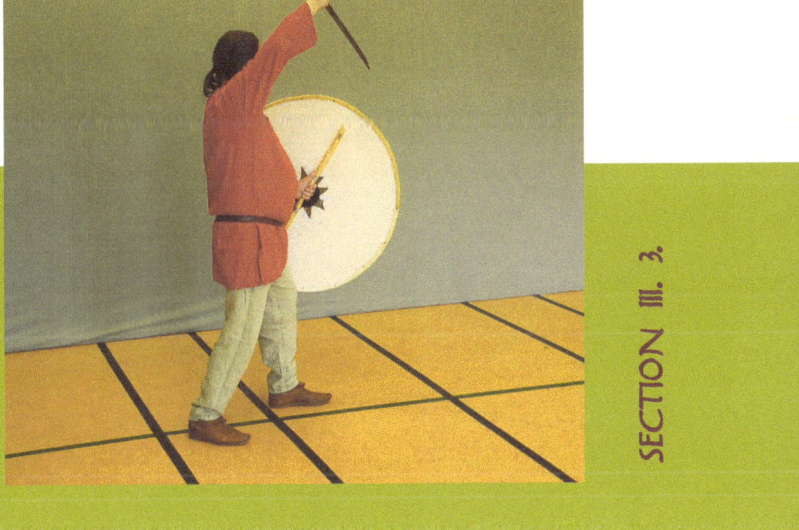

The sword is in an ideal position to counter attack after the parry.

The point is outside the left shoulder at about 45 degrees to straight ahead, and the hand is above the head.

Here we examine Ox on the left hand side, this time with the blade hanging down to the right side which is used to cover the right shoulder and head. This position is more awkward and dropping the point down further to defend lower targets is difficult.

We recommend this parry only to be used in an emergency situation, and if you wish to defend targets lower down turn the hand and use parry 4 from the first book. Used with care and always keeping the opponent in view, this position may be useful against left handed people.

This parry requires practise to find the correct angle and timing to be successful. The hand is slightly raised on contact so that the parry pushes into the attack, because this hand position is slightly biomechanically weaker than in the other single handed Ox.

SECTION III. 3.

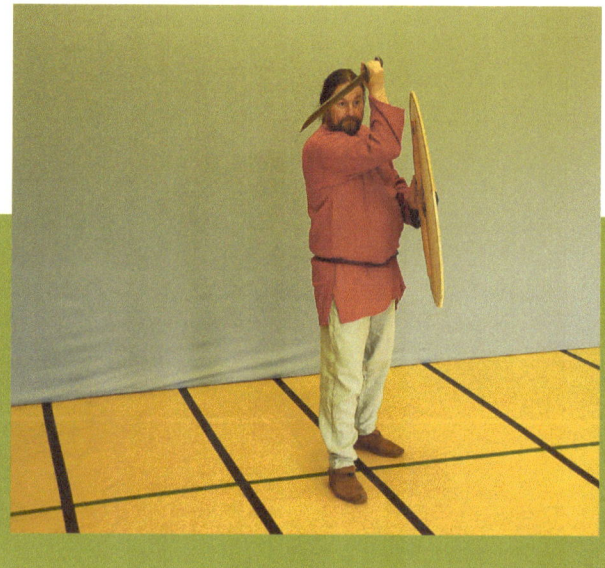

The sword point moves over and covers the high line, the head and right shoulder.

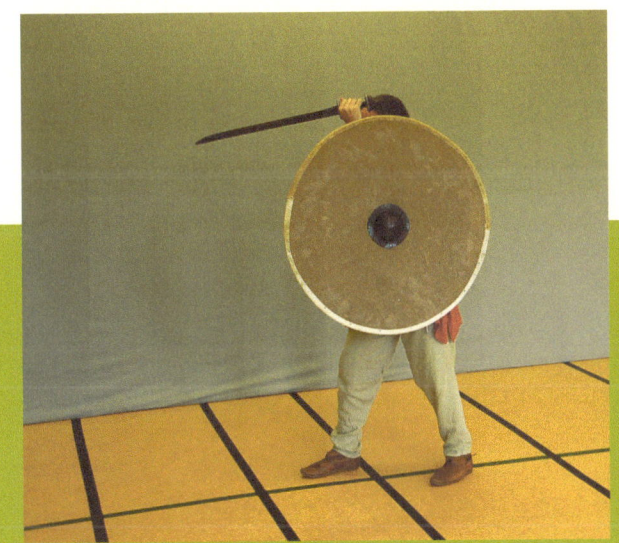
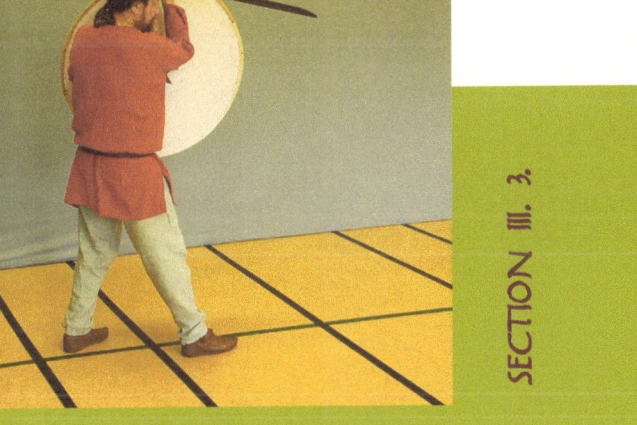

SECTION III. 3.

The sword is in an ideal position to counter attack after the parry.

The point is outside the right shoulder at about 45 degrees to straight ahead, and the hand is forward and above the head.

SECTION IV – USING SWORD AND SHIELD

THE CONCEPT OF INSIDE AND OUTSIDE LINE

When studying combat the concepts of inside and outside line are useful to know. An attacking line is usually a route to a part of the opponent's body from the object used to attack, such as high and low line. The centre line is an imaginary line used in the explanation of technique and movement in combat between two fighters. This line is drawn on diagrams connecting the two fighters' centres so that the geometry of the effect of movement can be better described. Subsidiary lines can be also added and used to describe other aspects of the positional relationship between the fighters.

Outside and inside lines deal with the position of the opponent's weapon or shield after contact with the opponent's weapon or shield relative to the body of the fighter. This will be treated in more depth in the advanced guides.

Generally after a parry if you can see the inside of the opponent's weapon arm, that is an inside parry. If you can see the back of the opponent's weapon arm you have made an outside parry. This situation is the same when applied to the shield side, if the opponent has parried with the shield face, then the sword lies on the outside. If the opponent has used the edge to parry or you can see the inside of

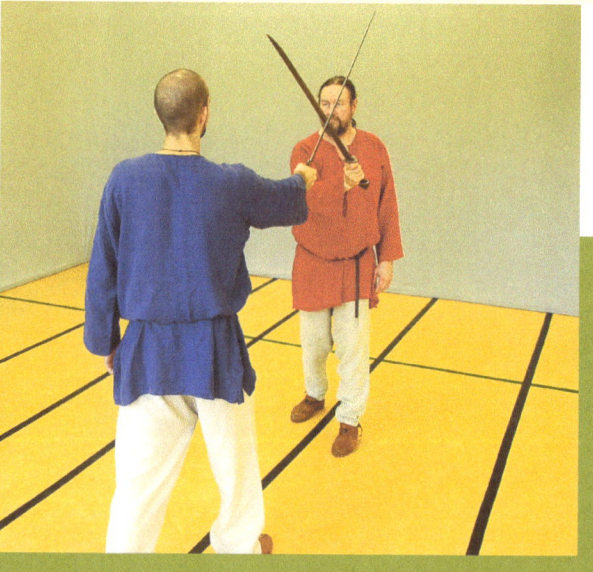

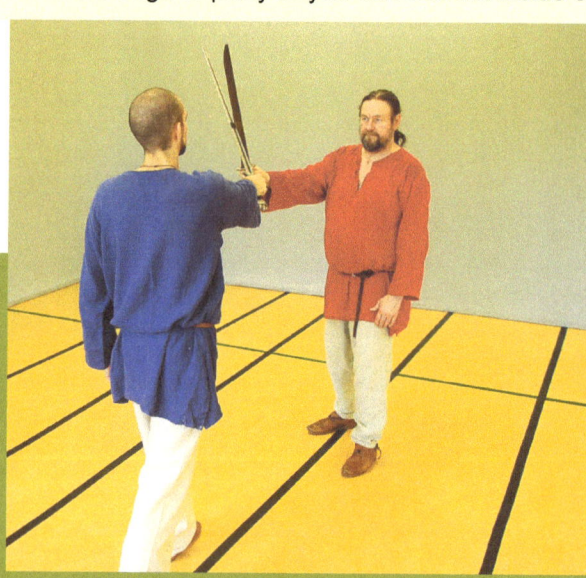

Red and Blue stand on the central line. Red's sword parry is on the inside. Blue's sword is also on the inside, even though Red has closed the line to the target and has the advantage. It does not matter if either sword point is up or down.

Both Red's sword and Blue's sword are on the outside though the advantage again lies with Red as he has closed the line to the target. It does not matter if either sword point is up or down.

the shield then usually you are on the inside. If the opponent's sword and shield are together and you had contact with the shield face and the sword at the same time, you would be outside to the shield and inside to the sword. In this case exploiting the inside position would be difficult as the shield would prevent this, so moving to the outside of either the shield or sword would be indicated.

Being inside or outside means there are different options available to the warrior in the counter attack phase of the fight. In general terms a preferred position is to be on the outside than on the inside though both have their advantages and disadvantages. Gaining the outside means that in the simplest terms, one of the arms of the opponent is partially blocked by the other. Being on the inside means that later movement can be either to the right or left, and the opponent generally has no idea which way you will go. The inside position also sometimes allows the possibility to attack through the middle of both defending weapons.

Please note that inside and outside positions depend upon the hand being used to make the contact. Right hand against right hand and left against left, both fighters are either inside or outside depending on the above. Right hand against left then the positions switch, one is inside the other is outside. Generally the position, either inside or outside can be exploited by using the technique called Exchanging the Parry. See next section.

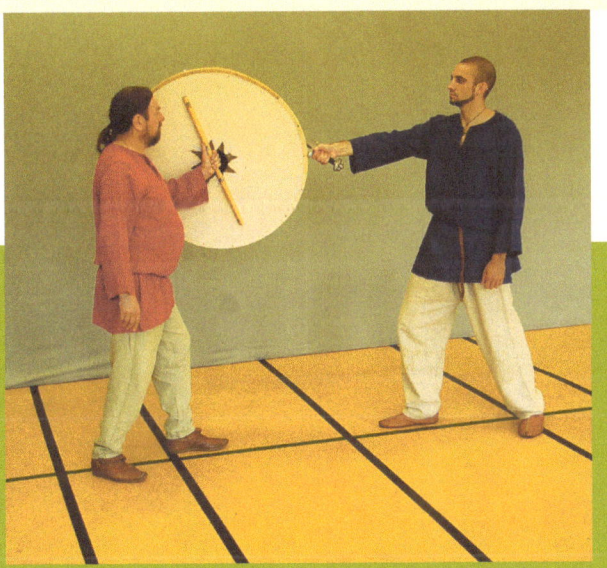

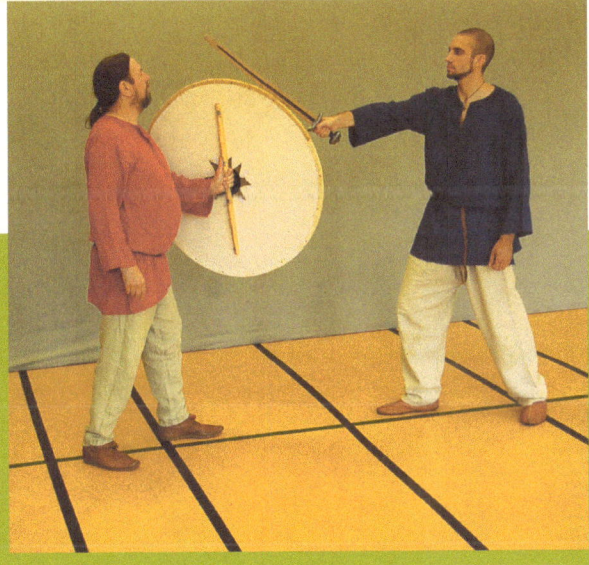

Red's shield parry is on the inside. Blue's sword is on the outside.

Red's shield parry is on the outside. Blue's sword is on the inside.

EXCHANGING THE PARRY

Sometimes an advantage can be created by parrying with a weapon that is not expected and then exchanging the parrying weapon, freeing up the original parrying weapon to continue the attack. This can create an opening by throwing the opponent's concentration off balance. A good example of this is parrying with the sword when the opponent expects the fighter to use the shield and then using the shield to exchange the parry from the sword. This mode of parrying also allows the fighter to swap from inside to outside or reversed, in situations where achieving the desired position would have been difficult in the first instance because of the initial movement of the opponent.

The roof parry is good for this type of manoeuvre as it slightly easier to swap from the inside to the outside because the sword does not obstruct the use of the shield.

The most important point about exchanging parries is the timing of the manoeuvre. The exchange must take place immediately after the parry and therefore the technique must be prepared by placing the shield close to the sword as it parries the opponent's weapon. In the 1.33 Treatise, the sword and buckler are positioned side by side, so that they are as close as possible. With larger shields close proximity is sometimes awkward, though the essence of the principle must be maintained, a quick exchange is essential for success.

In a real situation this control with the shield could be a hard hit with the aim of breaking the opponent's arm or fingers, thereby probably ending the fight. Using the shield as a weapon will be covered in later volumes.

Exchanging Shield for Sword
Here the sword is used to make an inside parry against attack 1 or 2, the sword is exchanged for the shield on the **outside**. Combined with stepping to the outside, this immediately off-sides the opponent's shield, making it very difficult to use to parry with. The larger the shield the more pronounced is the disadvantage. This opens up the whole right side of the opponent.

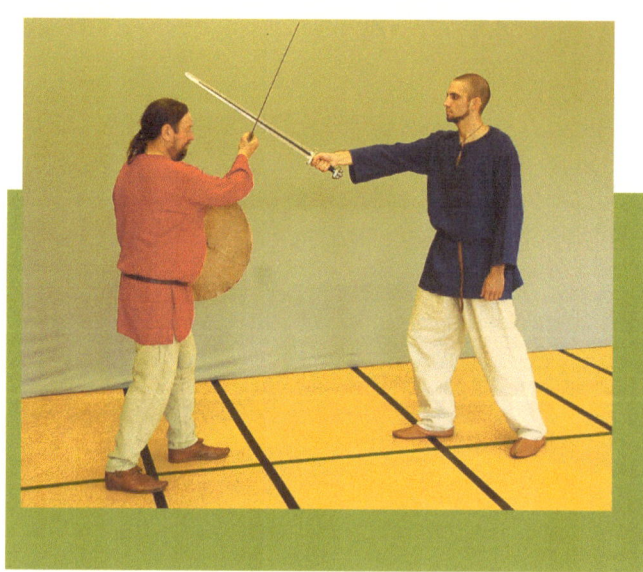

Red's sword has parried on the inside, against an attack to the shoulder or head.

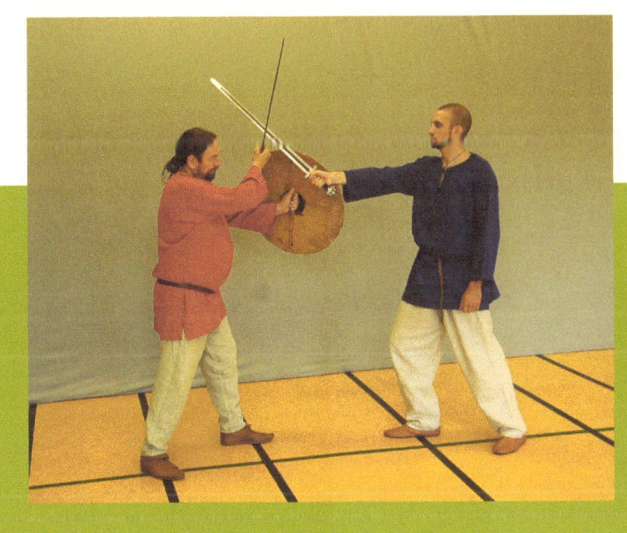 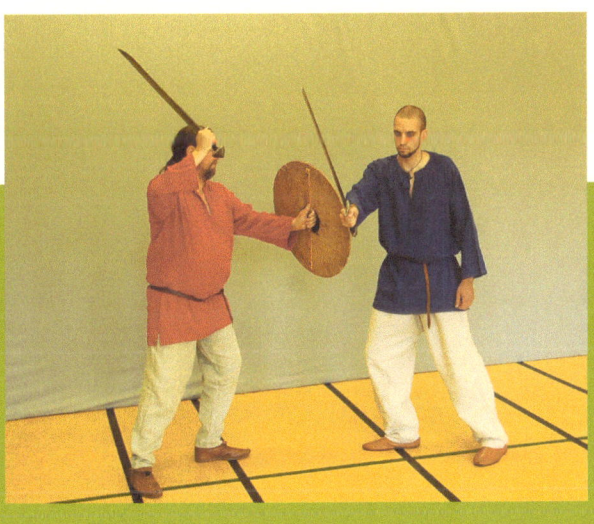

Red's shield has contacted the outside of Blue's weapon arm thereby taking control of the sword.

The exchange has taken place so that the sword is free to be used again.

Here the sword is used to make an inside parry against attack 1 or 2, the sword is exchanged for the shield on the **inside**.

The quickest target is usually the sword arm. If the opponent parries with the shield, this will present an excellent opportunity to use a combination strike. Such as attacking the left leg immediately after the attack to the arm, while stepping slightly diagonally forward to the right. Exchanging on the inside and moving to the right off-sides the opponent's weapon and makes it more difficult to counter attack, as the movement is away from their weapon and the shield is interposed in the correct position. We will explore this in more detail in the Partner Drills section.

SECTION IV. 2.

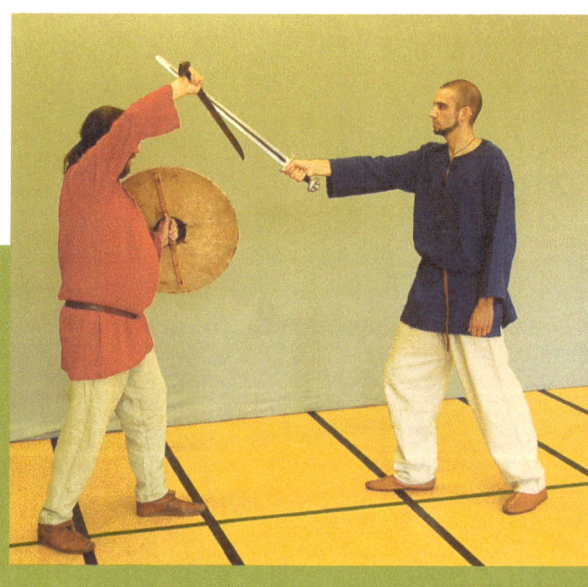

Red's sword has parried on the inside with the point down, against an attack to the shoulder or head

Summary for Exchanging the Parry

- The shield must be in close proximity to the sword
- The exchange must be made immediately after the parry
- Basically the timing of the move is everything
- Outside exchanges are usually more difficult to survive than inside exchanges
- The inside exchange allows the possibility of striking between the opponent's sword and shield
- From the inside the fighter can go left or right in subsequent movements easier than on the outside

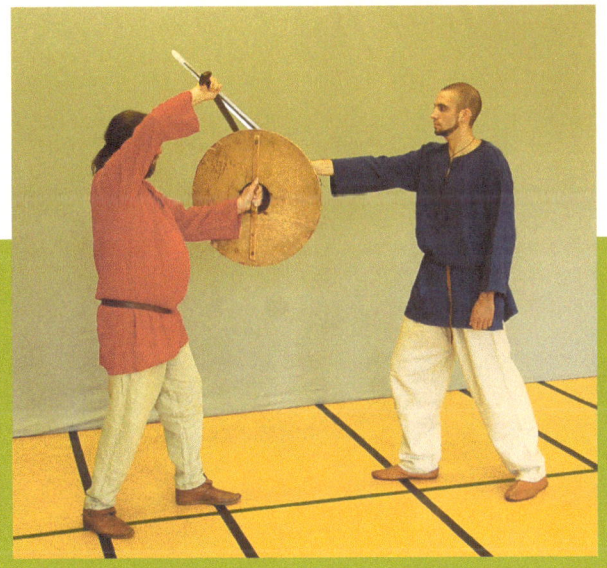

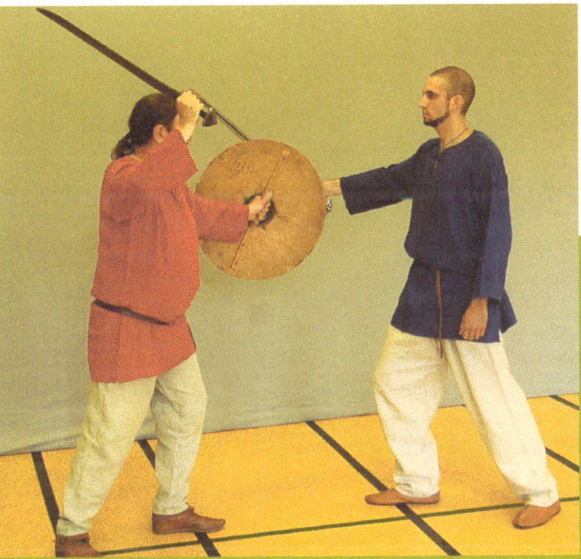

Red's shield has contacted the inside of Blue's sword thereby taking control of the sword.

The exchange has taken place so that the sword is free to be used again.

DISARMING THE WEAPON

This is a complicated subject though some of the more basic disarming techniques are easy to learn and put into practice. Most of these techniques that we will cover are based on either a pommel grab or a blade grab. We present two, though they both require the use of the shield hand, so normally they are only performed when you have lost your shield or you drop it at the right moment to surprise your opponent.

Disarm Using the Pommel Grab
This disarm is probably the most common one practised, because it is extremely effective. It is possible to do this from sword parry 2, though then the free hand goes over the sword arm, on the outside of the blade.

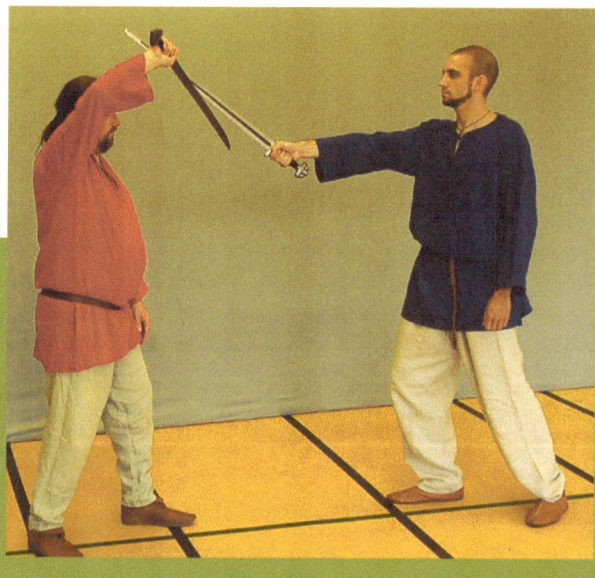

Red uses the roof block in the right ox guard to parry the weapon.

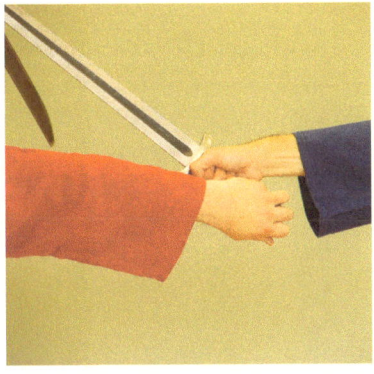

Here is a close up of the hands, note the grip on the pommel.

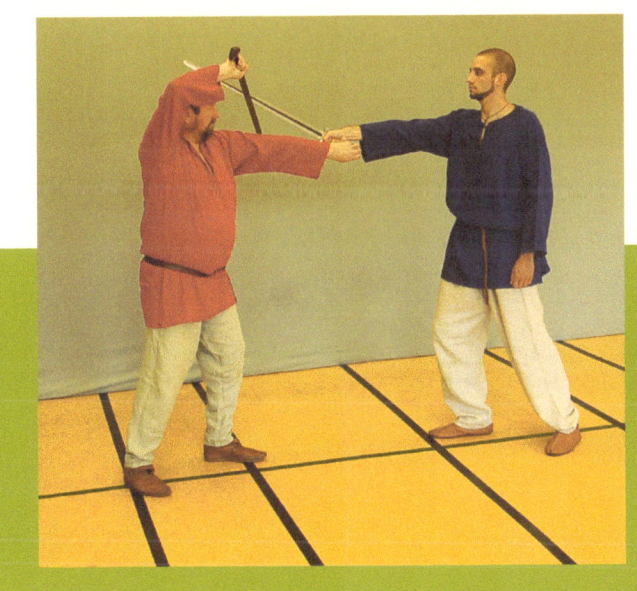

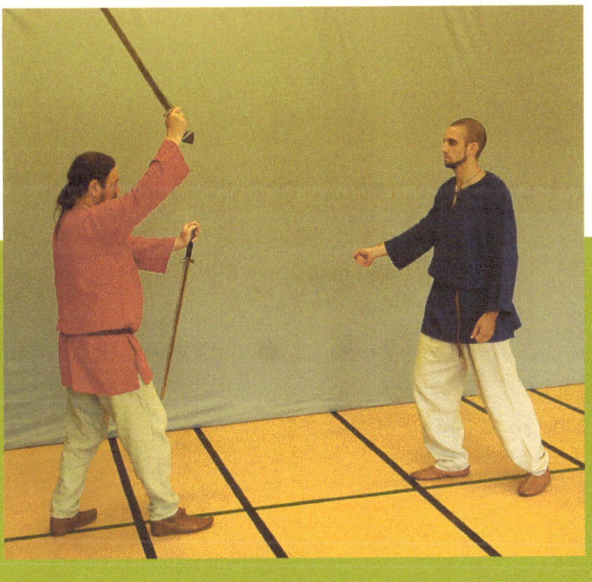

Pass under the sword with the left hand, using a half step if needed, and grab the opponent's pommel.

Pull the pommel towards you while making a full step backward.

Disarm Using the Blade Grab Near the Grip

If the rules you fight to allow the blade to be gripped, then this is another easy method to remove the opponent's weapon! Of course in a real fight with sharp weapons, with or without gloves, this is still possible. As long as the blade does not move in the hand, it should not cut. The action of grabbing the blade of sharp weapons is fairly common in medieval combat treatises. Medieval swords are believed to have been fairly blunt near the grip. You can also adopt to grab the blade only with the fingers on the flat sides.

In this situation it would also be possible to grab the pommel though this would require a small step and therefore slightly more time. Also the sword would come out of the back of the hand in the same manner as the blade grab.

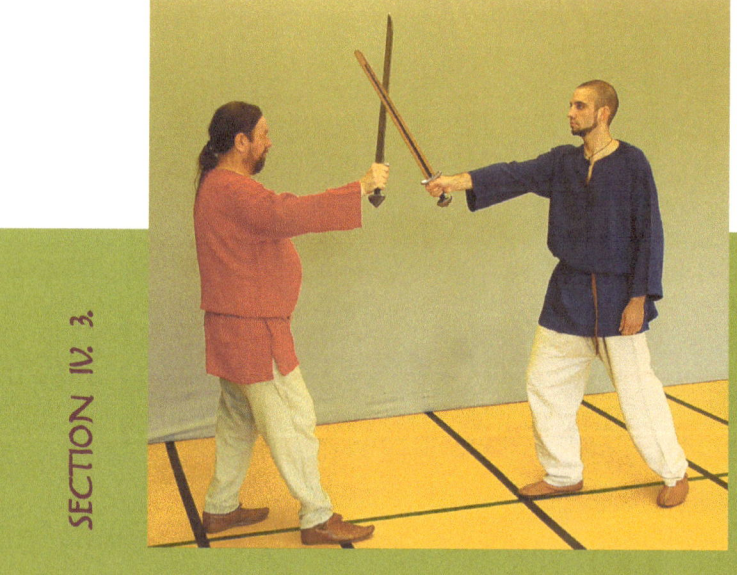

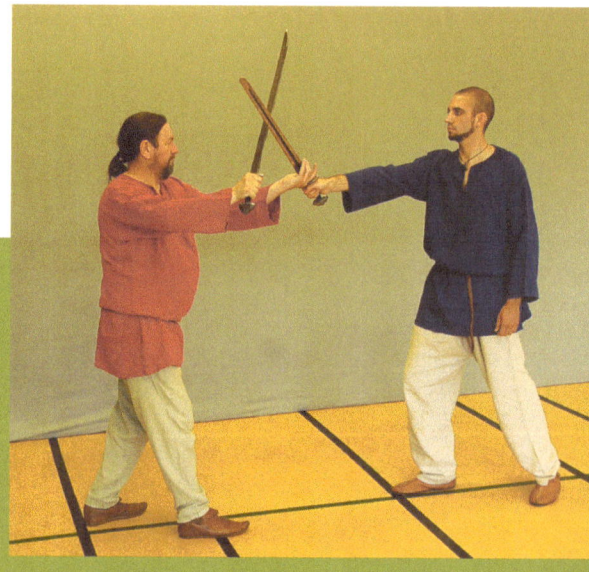

Red uses the outside parry to parry the weapon.

Red using the left hand, grips Blue's sword blade with the thumb pointing to the left, palm up.

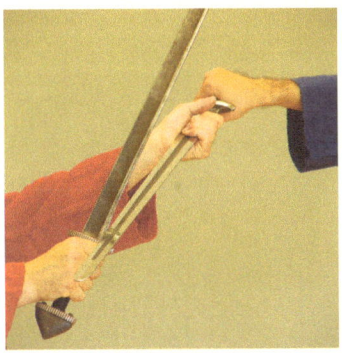

Here is a close up of the hands later in the turn, note the grip on the blade.

Summary for Disarming the Weapon

- One hand must be empty at the time of disarming
- The opponent's sword must be fixed at the moment of disarm, usually with a parry
- The force can be increased by pushing the opponent's blade with the sword
- The power of the move is greatly increased by stepping away at the point of disarming
- Any point on the blade can be grabbed to disarm
- The pommel is an ideal place to grab to make a disarm

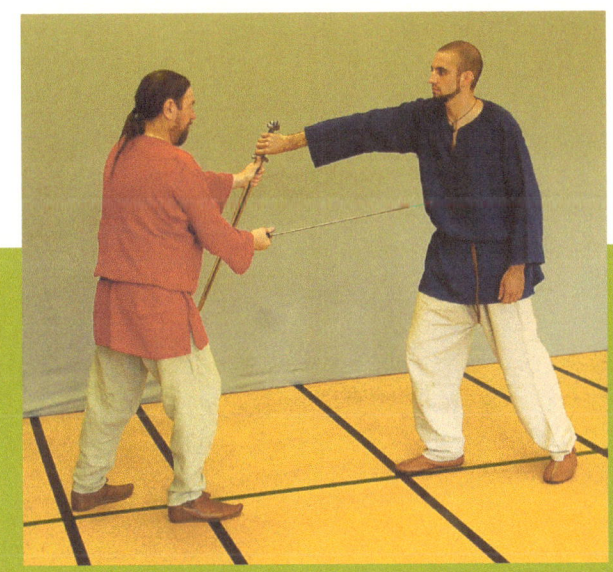

Red pulls downward, turning Blue's sword point to the floor, the turn is made until the sword is released. Red can assist with this move by also turning his own sword downward, this might even cut the opponent as the motion is made.

SECTION IV. 3.

SECTION V – SINGLE PERSON DRILLS

SWORD HAND PROTECTION USING THE SHIELD

Drills 1-10

This drill addresses the real problem of hand protection when using the Viking period sword with its small cross guard. The cross guard does nothing to protect the hand while you attack. When fighting with rules that allow a full body target this is a useful skill to learn. This is also exactly what the Vikings themselves had to do! Of course if you know where the opponent's sword is, because he has just attacked you, then the protection of the sword hand is not so urgent. The sword hand is protected by the edge of the shield. With a large shield some protection will be afforded to the rest of the body even while it defends the hand. Smaller shields can usually only do one job.

Obviously if the cut goes through the object or misses the target the fighter could end in one of the other guard positions. Even so at the position of maximum reach the hand will be exposed unless the shield is used as shown. Try cutting from each of the basic guard positions and end up in the same positions as shown below. You should train both attacks and parries so that you can automatically end in a position with a protected hand.

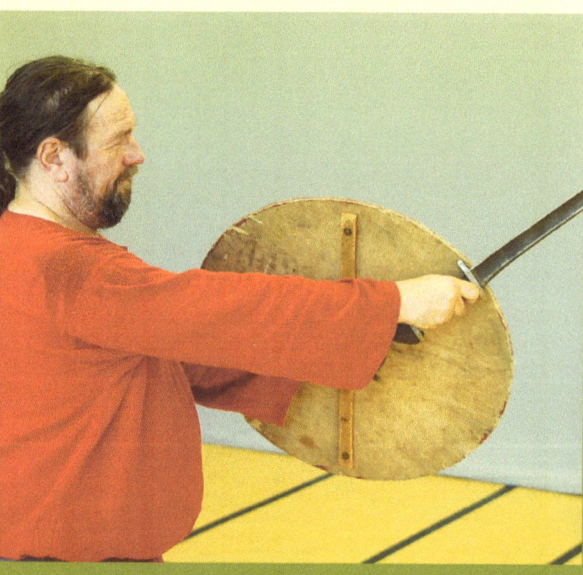

Drill 1

Attack to Head
After an attack to the opponent's head. The weapon hand is still protected at contact.

Right Handed
The first 5 positions are from the **right** hander's perspective.

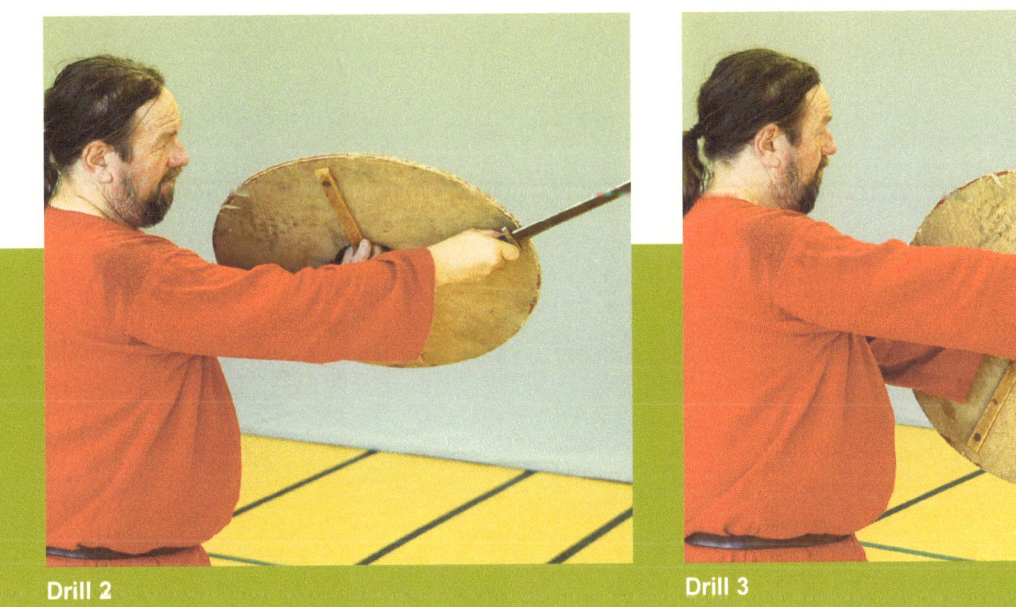

Drill 2

Drill 3

Attack to the Left Shoulder
When striking with the sword from the right shoulder or head. This is the most common attack from a right hander.

Attack to the Right Shoulder
When striking with the sword from the left shoulder. Likewise this is the most common attack from a left hander.

> **Important!**
> We show this drill from both the right hander's and the left hander's perspective. Make sure you train the one you need for your style of fighting.

SECTION V.1.

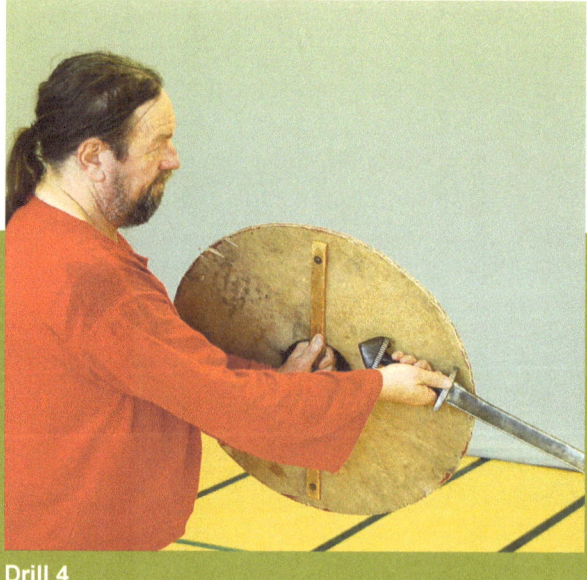

Drill 4

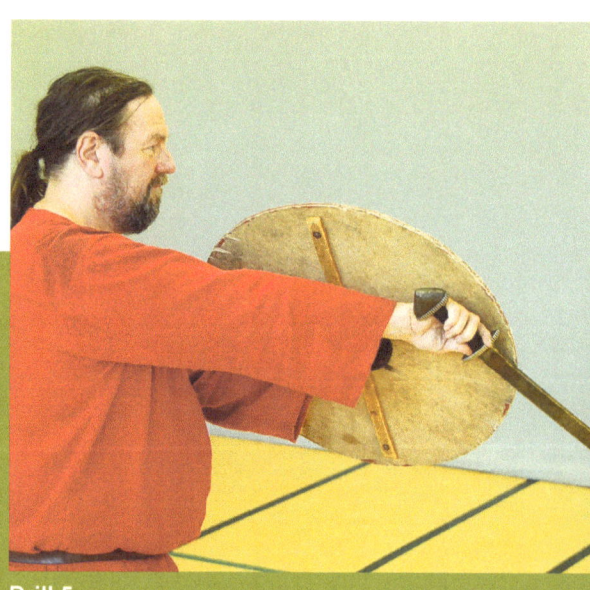

Drill 5

Attack to the Left Hip
When striking with the sword from the right hip.

Attack to the Right Hip
When striking with the sword from the left hip.

Left Hander

This series of pictures shows how to protect the hand with the shield while using the sword in the left hand. This is a mirror image of the right hander's perspective.

This also means that the most powerful attack from a left hander comes in towards the right shoulder or head of the right handed opponent. This is also the unshielded side. The same situation applies to the left hander attacked by the right hander.

Even if the rule set that you use does not allow hand hits it is very good practice to defend against them, because the hand and fingers are easily damaged and can take a long time to heal. Accidental hits can be just as debilitating as aimed hits, so in the end it pays to defend the yourself as best you can regardless of the rules used.

Understanding the subtle differences between hand positions after cuts and thrusts, can be useful in creating tactical sequences. This subject will be expanded in later guides.

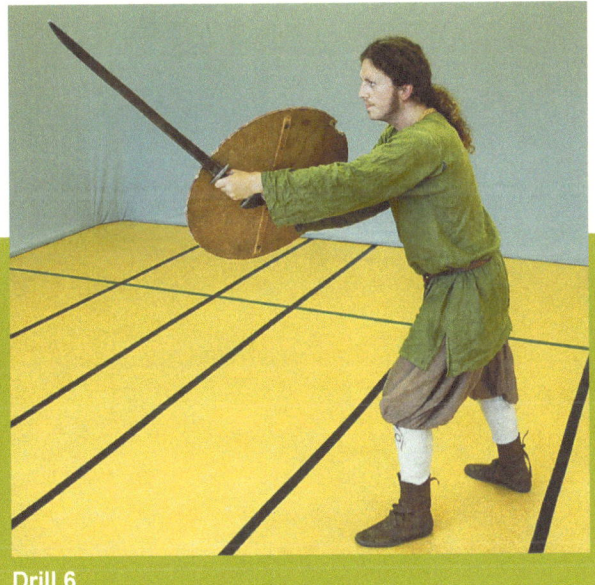

Drill 6

Attack to Head
After an attack to the opponent's head. The weapon hand is still protected at contact.

SECTION V. 1.

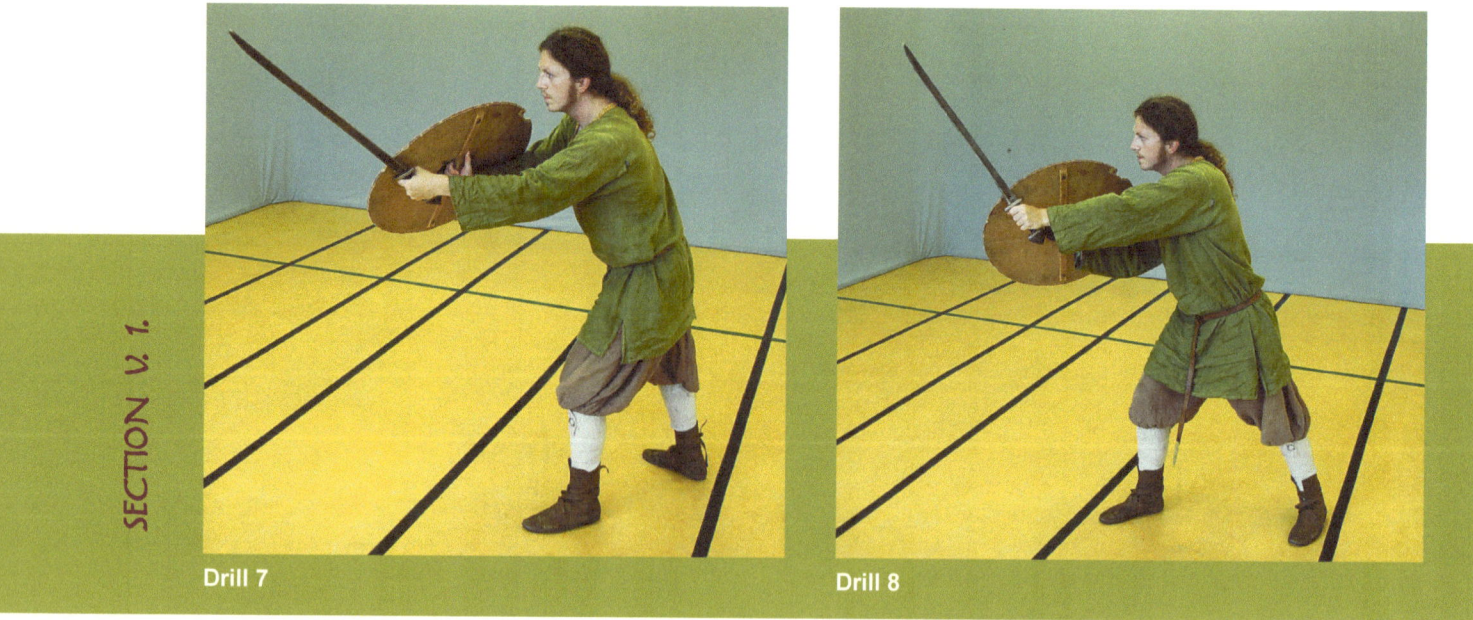

Drill 7

Drill 8

Attack to the Right Shoulder
When striking with the sword from the left shoulder. This is the most common attack from a left hander.

Attack to the Left Shoulder
When striking with the sword from the right shoulder. This is not often used by the left hander.

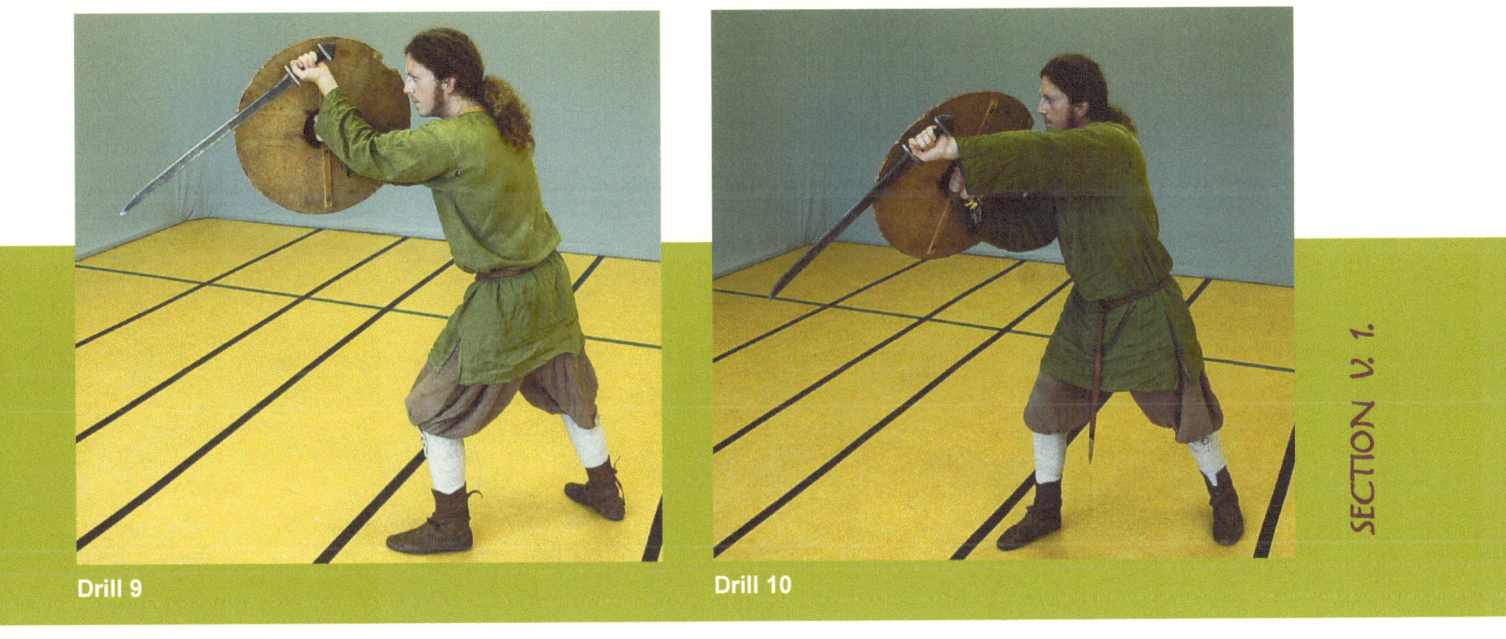

Drill 9

Drill 10

Attack to the Right Hip or Right Under Arm
When striking with the sword from the left hip. This is a common attack from a left hander.

Attack to the Left Hip or Left Under Arm
When striking with the sword from the right hip.

VARYING STRIKING ANGLES AGAINST THE PELL

Drills 11-12

This simple drill demonstrates that the angle and therefore the target of cuts from above and below can be varied. In our first volume, we made three attacks from above and two from below. The purpose of this drill is to show that in certain circumstances all targets can be attacked from above, by just altering the angle of cut to the target. So an attack to the shoulder can be altered to an attack to an exposed thigh.

Likewise most cuts from below can target upper body areas with an alteration of attack angle or even angle of step. A cut under the shield edge can target as high up as the arm pit, not just the thigh.

Varying strike angle is just another aspect of control of the weapon. Knowing how to vary angle of trajectory leads to some interesting possibilities in our ability to defeat the opponent's defence when combined with footwork. In the advanced guides, this subject will receive much more attention when we explore the effect of attack angle and geometry. This is quite a large section and requires careful study.

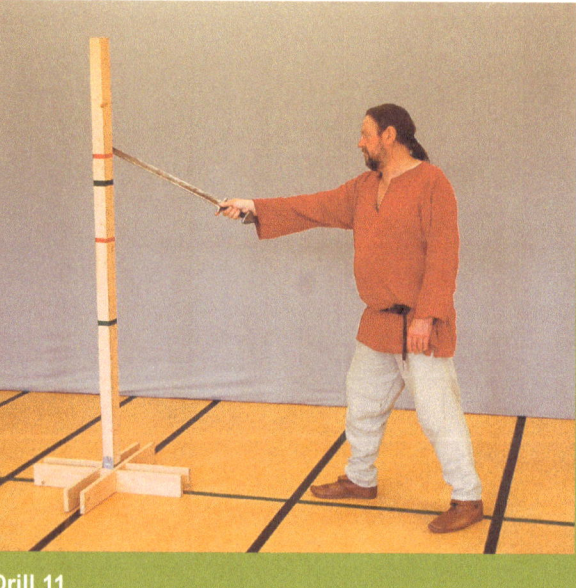

Drill 11

We start this drill with the normal cut from above targeting the shoulder. The change of angle in the cut is simple to do and can be learnt quickly. An alteration in angle can confuse the defender as to target of the cut if you wait to change the angle late in the swing.

Drill 11
Cut to the Thigh from Above.
This is especially useful if the opponent is in the process of raising the shield to defend against the high attack angle, altering the sword trajectory to travel across the face of the shield into the now exposed thigh.

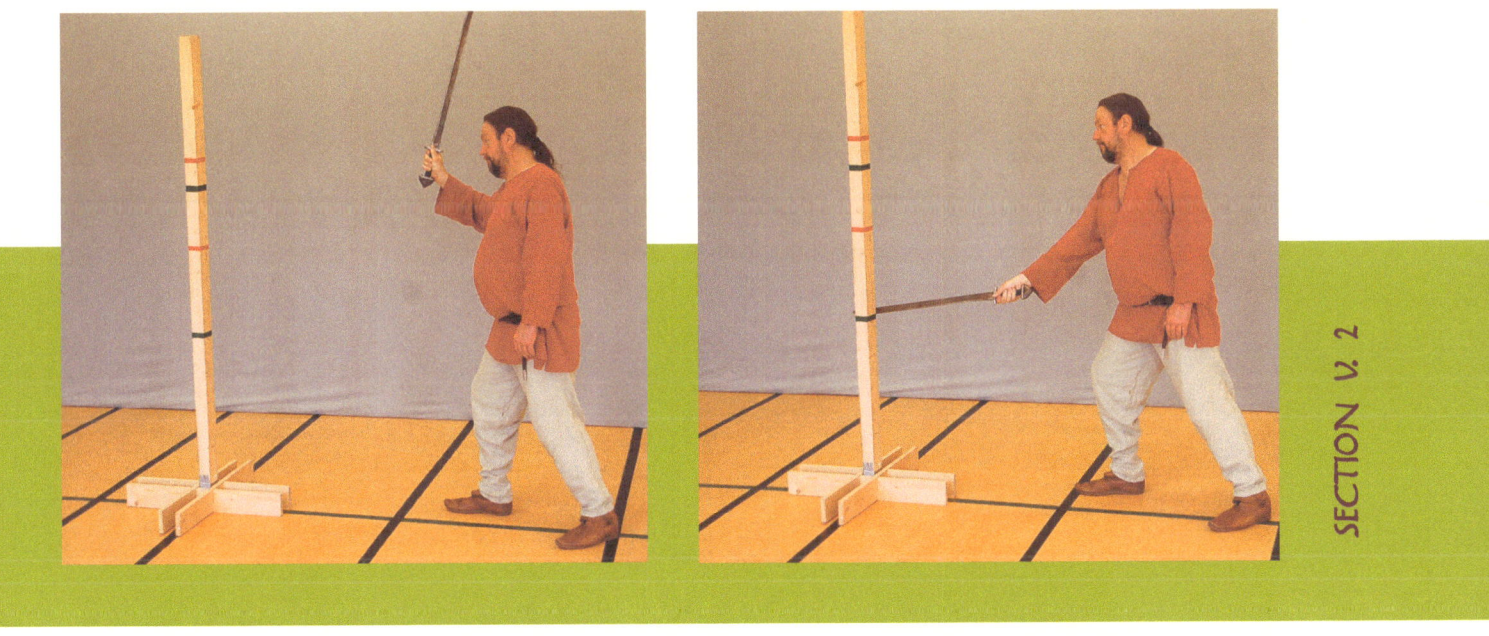

This is the transition picture, pulling back to make the attack to the thigh from above.

This picture shows the result of the modification of the angle to cut the thigh from above. This cut can travel down across the face of the shield, the opponent unaware that his leg is exposed.

Drill 12
Cut to the Arm Pit or Arm from Below
This is an excellent variation to the under cut against the thigh. This can be used against people using two weapons, small shields or large shields, by stepping off line to either side other targets open up.

By going to the opponent's left, his side and shoulder may be open; going to the opponent's right you can cut right under the shield up to the left armpit or chest.

Using the other cut from below on the other side, attack no. 5 can be used to cut between the sword arm and the shield rim up into the right arm pit or the chest or even the stomach area.

Also if the attack was against the thigh and was blocked with the sword using parry 5, the attack can be continued by taking off the sword from the bind and attack the upper sword arm with a cut from below.

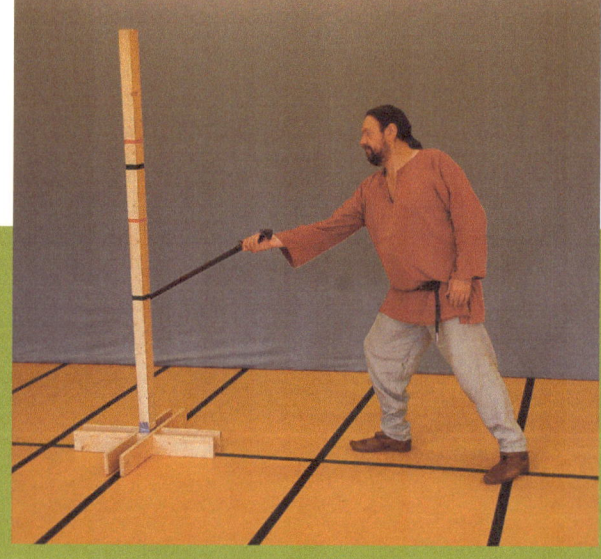

Drill 12

This shows the normal cut from below to a thigh level target. Remember this could be lower down the leg as well, though then the fighter would have to lower his stance by bending the knees.

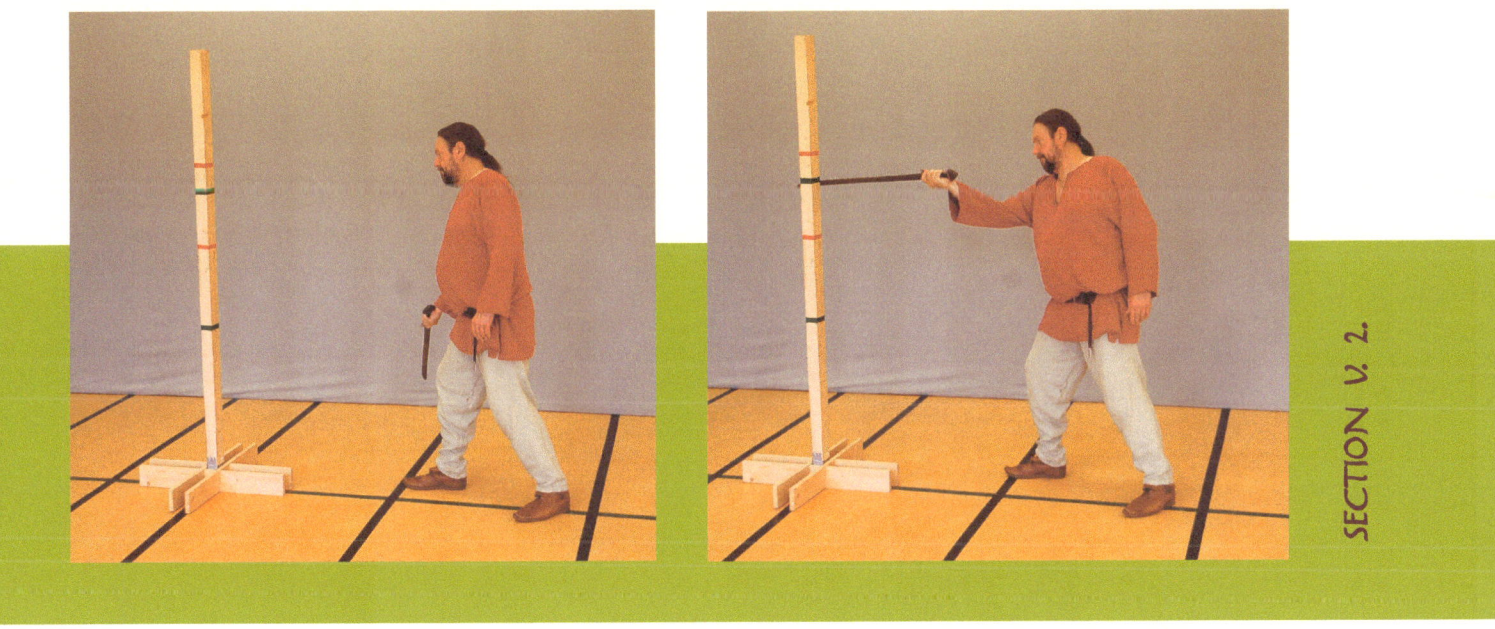

This is the transition picture, pulling back to make the attack to the arm pit level target.

This cut from below targets the arm pit, and in some circumstances it can come up underneath the shield, or possibly outside the edge of the shield. By orientating the cut more to the left it can target the weapon arm as an attack comes in. This is a very useful counter attack, which is often hard to see.

COMBINATION STRIKES USING DIAGONAL HALF STEPS AGAINST THE PELL

Drills 13-20

After establishing a good position for the pell so that you can step all around it on all sides, practice the following two drill groups. This first group of drills is designed to facilitate learning of two strikes in combination with firstly a full step straight forward and then stepping to the side with a half step. Using two strikes to two widely spaced targets is a common approach, inducing the opponent to overreact to the first attack so that the second is successful.

Remember never look to the target you are going to next as people can learn to read your face.

In each drill the targets will be indicated in the text. Please feel free, once you are familiar with the concept to vary the target and the type of attack used to strike it. The second group of drills will use firstly a half step straight forward and then stepping to the side with a full step.

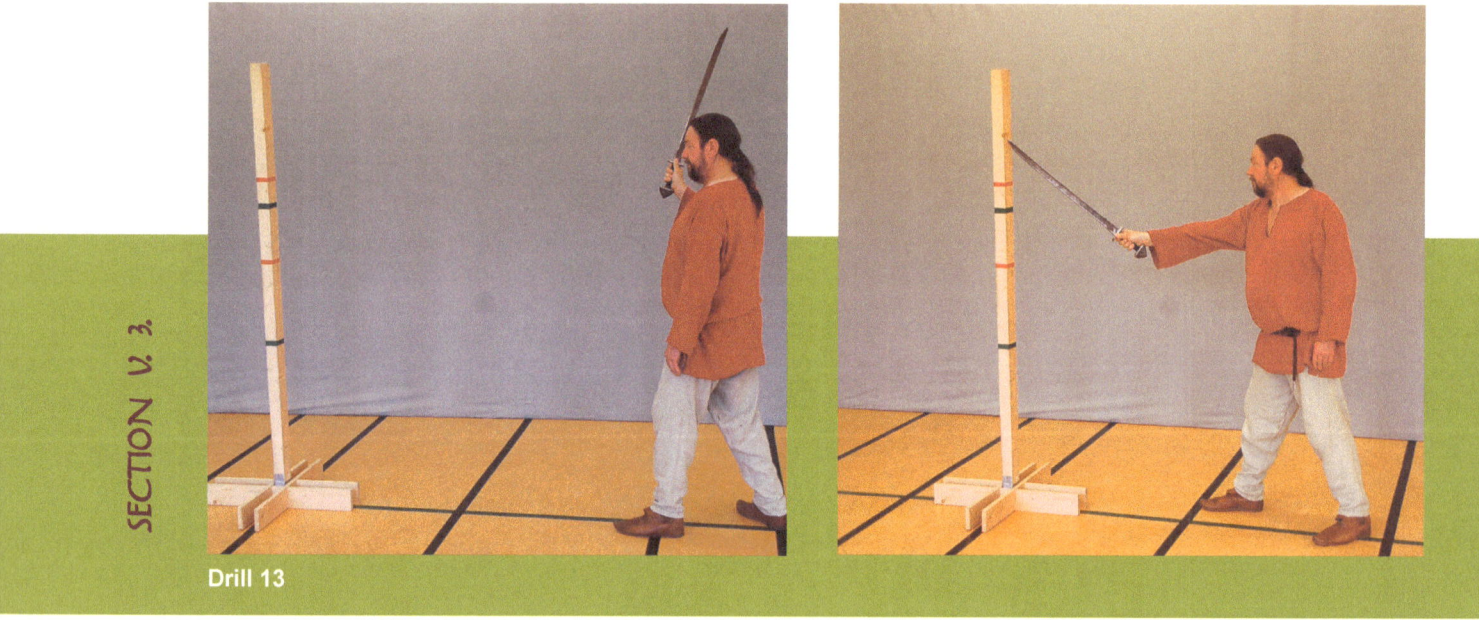

Drill 13

Red starts in guard position 1. To reach this position Red calibrates the distance by placing the sword on the target as if a full cut has been made and stepping back a full step. Initially Red strikes to the head with a full step forward; followed by striking to the left leg using a half step. This combination brings the opponent's shield high opening up the thigh on the shield side.

Red makes a full step and strikes to the head, this will initiate the first defensive action from the opponent.

Once you have mastered the basic movements and strikes without the shield repeat the drills while holding your own shield, always trying to imagine which is the most likely attack the opponent could make. Position the shield so that it will cover the part of your body which is closest to the opponent's weapon. This is usually covering the high line on the left or your weapon arm.

These manoeuvres are the core of basic tactics and therefore are extremely important to understand and learn. It is the interplay of stepping with the sequence of cuts that determine the flow of the fight. By continuous combinations the fighter can keep the initiative, destroy their psychological resistance, and overwhelm the opponent's defence.

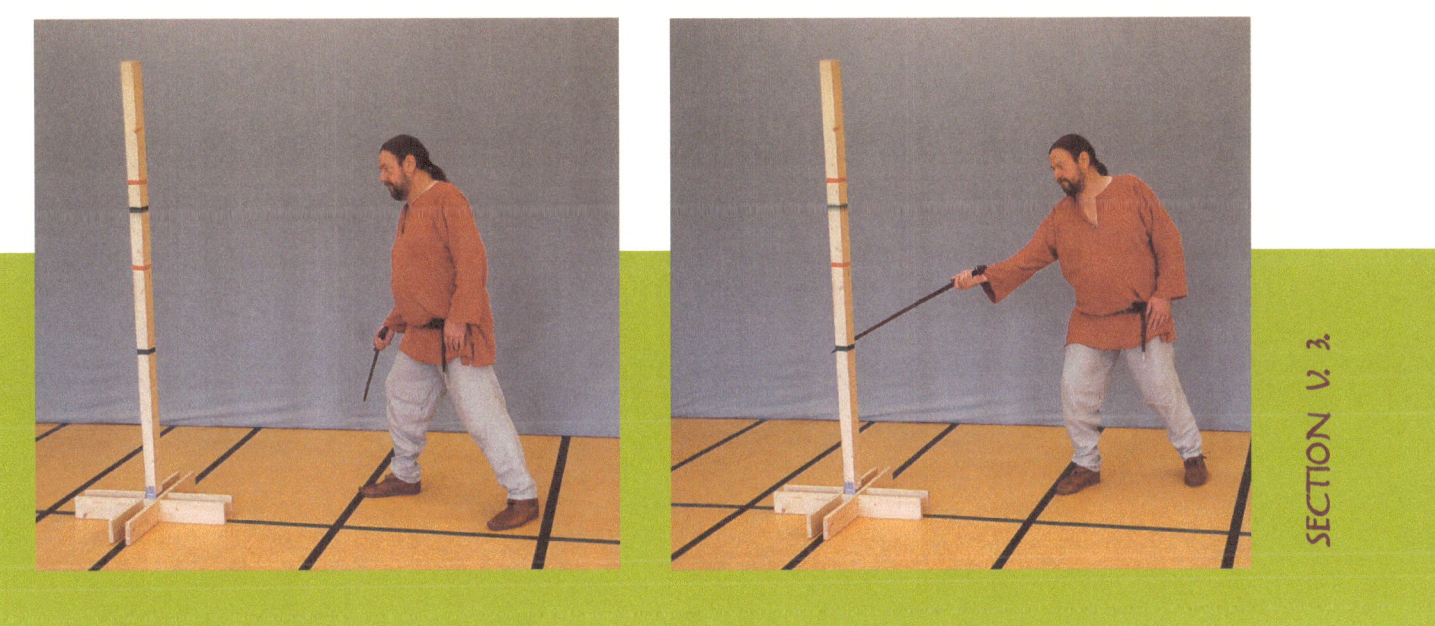

Red then makes a diagonal half step to the right; this will expose more of the target and also move away from the opponent's weapon.

Red executes a cut from below against the left leg. If the opponent is quick and has dropped the shield down to defend the leg, Red can then switch the attack again to the left shoulder with an attack from above.

Drill 14
Initially striking to the right shoulder with a full step, secondly striking to the left shoulder with a half step to the right.

Likewise this brings the opponent's shield over to his right with the first attack, and then swapping to the other shoulder as you go to the right. If the opponent protects the left shoulder quickly with the shield but stays high, the attack can be changed to quickly strike down to the left leg from above instead.

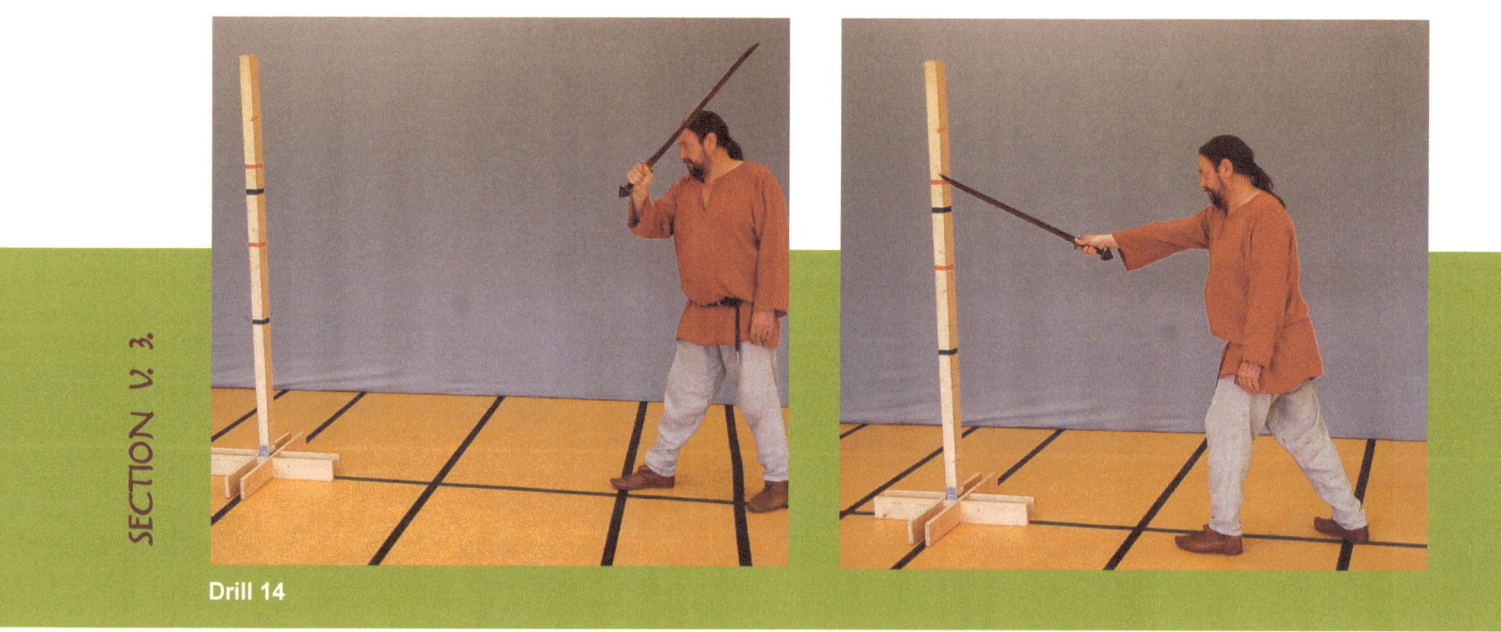

Drill 14

Starts in guard position 3 after calibration.

Red makes a full step with the left leg, and strikes to the left shoulder.

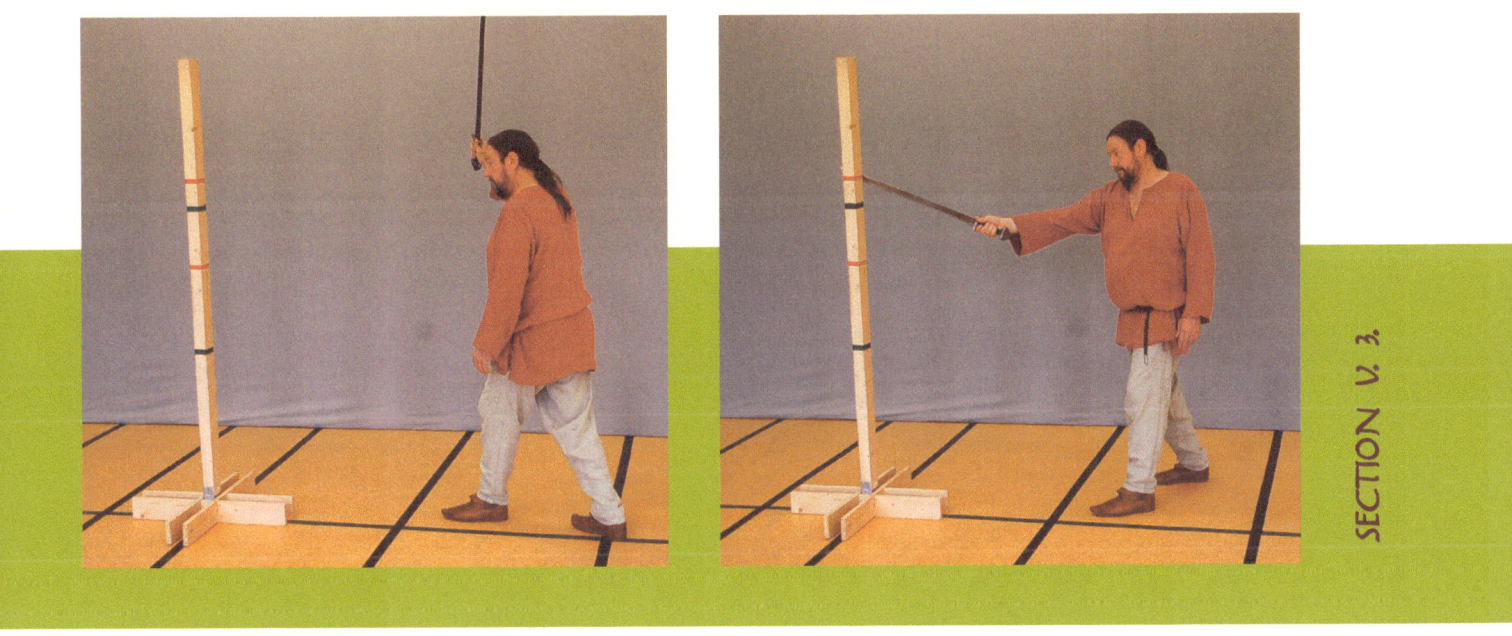

Red uses a diagonal half step to the right, with the left leg, Red's shield would be covering the high line, which if the opponent's weapon is high, is the shortest route to the target. If the opponent's weapon is low already, then the shield would be positioned to cover the low line.

Red then cuts against the left shoulder using attack 2. Having moved away from the opponent's weapon side, this position is relatively safe. Note Red has orientated his body to the target.

**Drill 15
Begin striking to the left leg from below using a full step, followed by a strike to the right shoulder utilising a half step to the left.**

This is a fairly common combination, and is tactically sound as long as you do not allow him to exchange parries if he blocks the second parry with the sword. See the next drill for a variation at the point of the start of the second attack. The main idea of this combination is to move the shield down and out to the opponent's left and then swap to attack high on the right, diagonally as far away from the shield as possible, while maintaining the sword side to the opponent, which will maximise your reach.

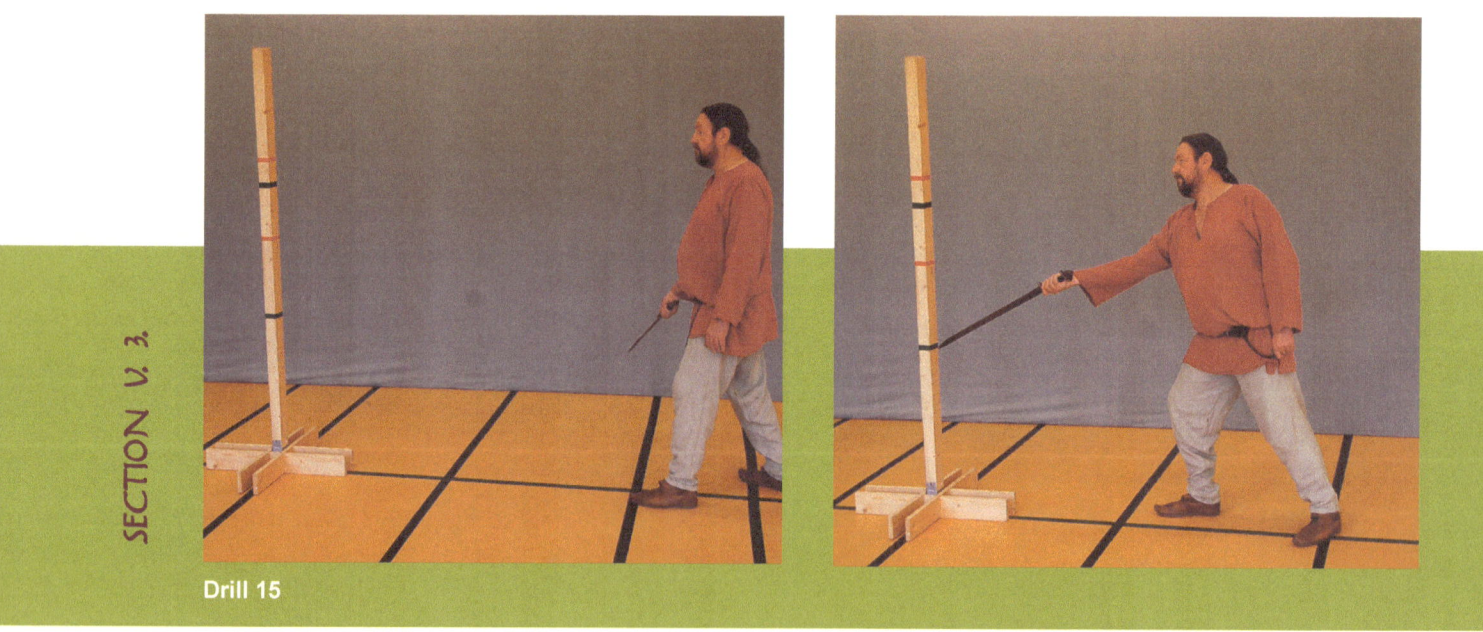

Drill 15

Red starts in guard position 4.

Red uses a full step and strikes to the left leg from below.

Careful positioning of the shield is essential for this type of manoeuvre. The shield must be very near and behind the sword at the end of the move, because if he parries with the second attack with the sword with parry 3, the attack can be continued by exchanging shield for sword on the outside at that point. The shield will also be in the best place to prevent a point down attack to the outside of the sword arm.

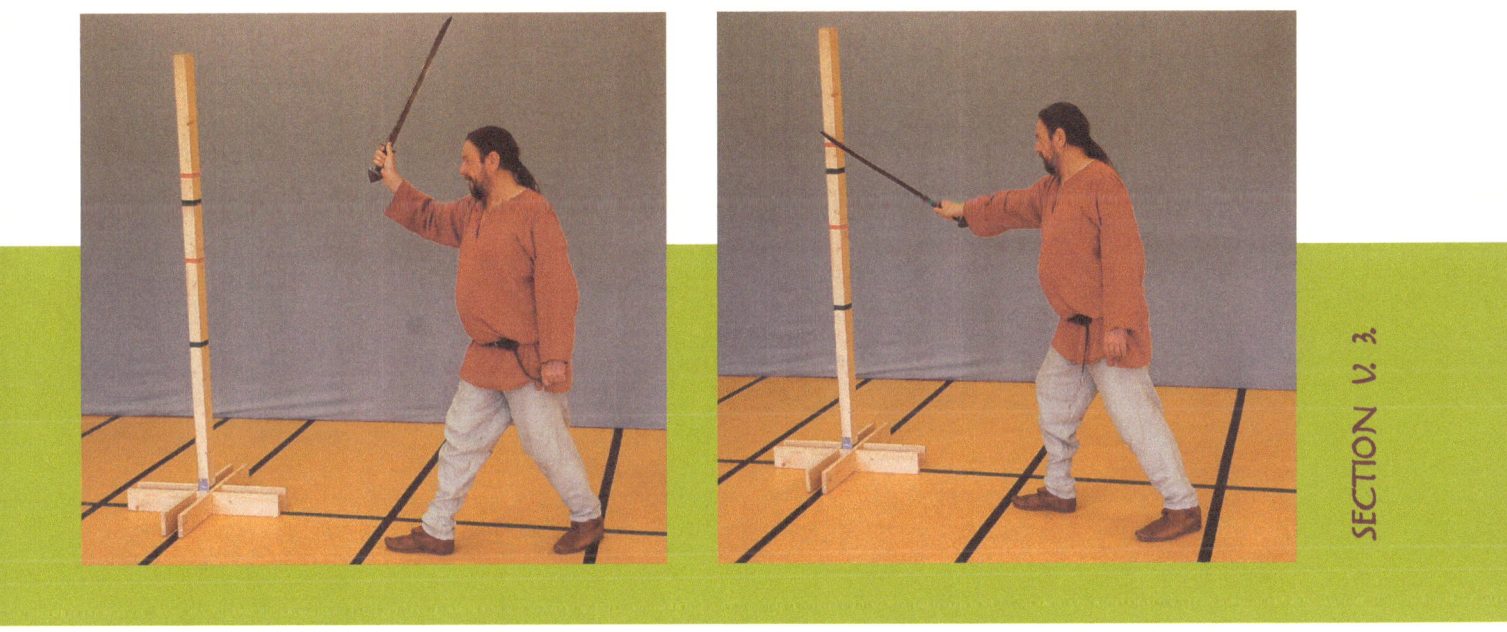

Making a diagonal half step to the right, brings Red closer to the unshielded side. Red's shield would cover the movement of the sword arm by close proximity, closing the attack lines of the opponent's sword.

Red then cuts to the right shoulder. This combination is also very useful if the opponent has attacked during the time between the first attack and the second. Normally this attack will expose his sword arm, allowing a switch from shoulder to arm, a much easier target to hit.

Drill 16
Initially striking to the left leg followed by an attack to the other leg using a half step.

This is an unusual combination and involves a transition from one low target to the other. Refer to drill 10. This is a variation at the point of choosing a target for the second attack. Remember not to bother striking to a target that is already covered. You have to develop a feeling for what is and is not possible in every position. The main point of such combinations is the surprise value, if the opponent is convinced that the second strike is going to the right shoulder, and you quickly change to strike the right leg. This sort of transition must be practised.

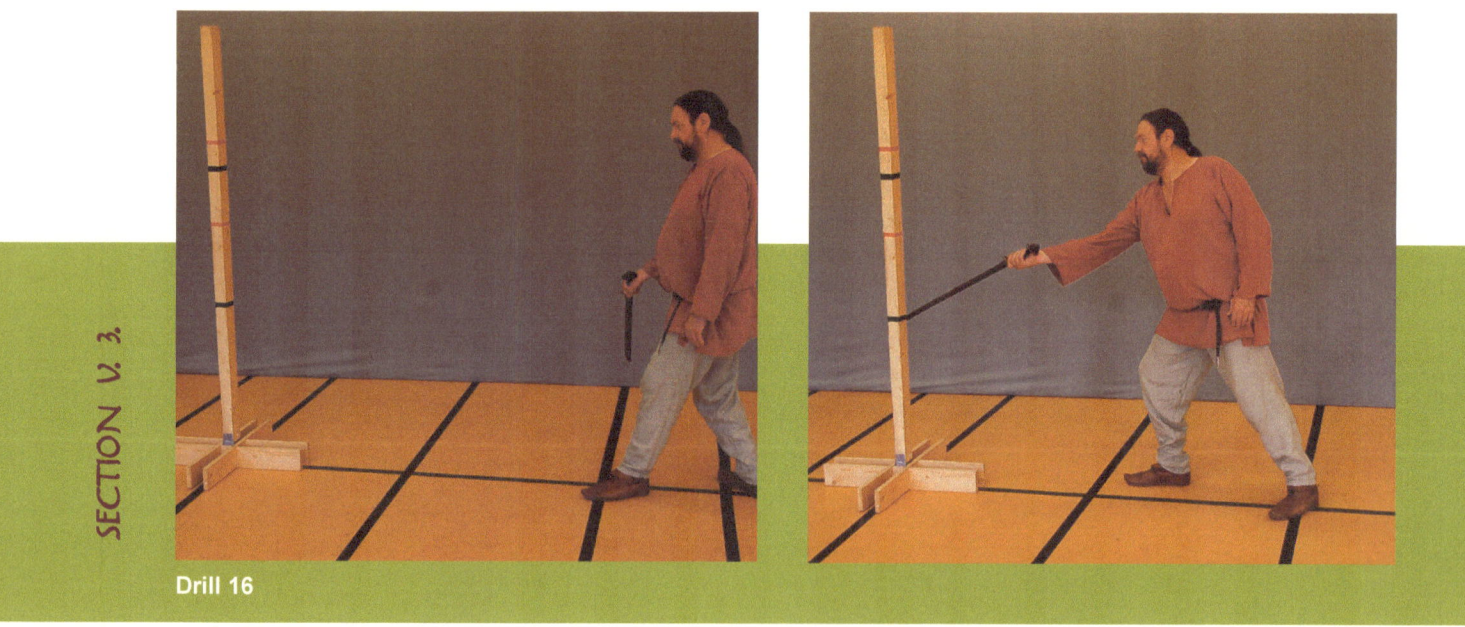

Drill 16

Red starts in guard position 4.

Red makes a full step and cuts from below to the left leg.

Remember if the opponent's sword is not committed elsewhere, the transition of the sword arm to the second attack has to be covered with the shield, this takes practice and requires good timing. The shield comes from behind your own sword as it falls to attack the leg and covers the opponent's attacking possibilities either by close proximity or by contact with his sword.

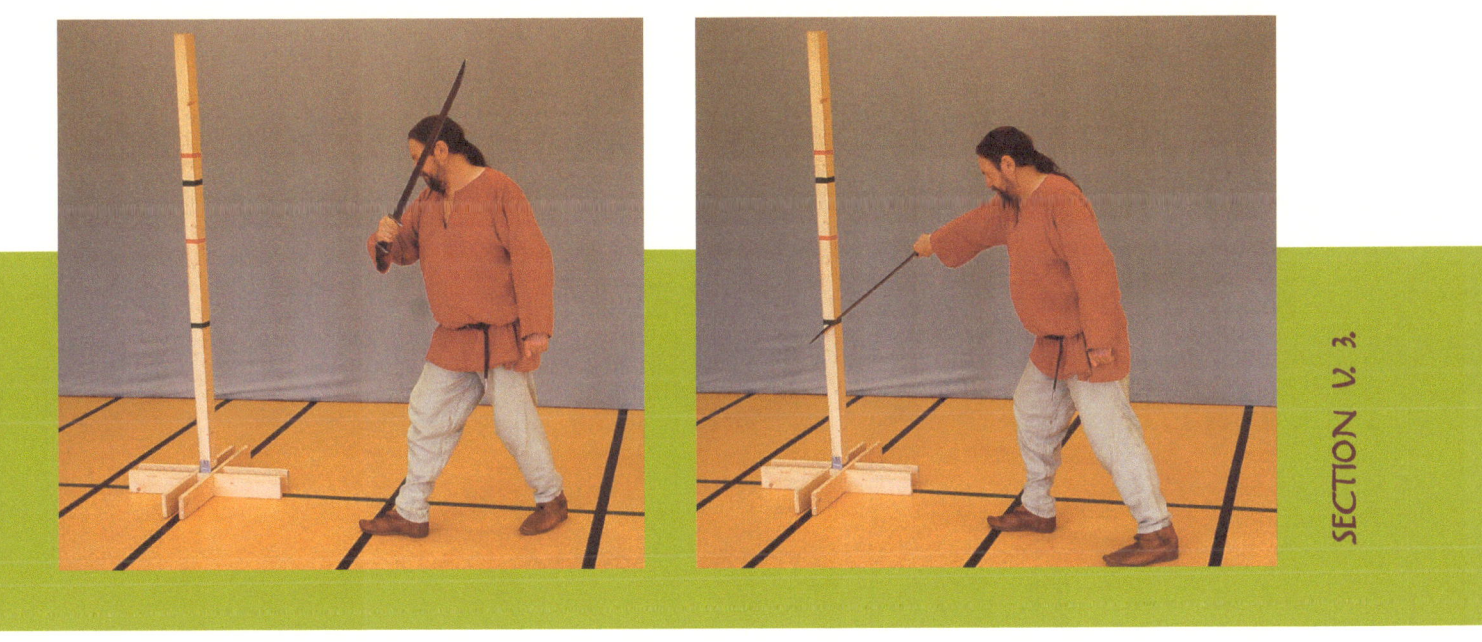

Red uses a diagonal half step to the left. The side step should be made quickly, immediately after the first attack has landed.

Red then cuts to the right leg with attack 5.
Before this attack can hit you may have had to engage the sword with the shield on the high line to make space for your sword to make the transition and the attack. This forward use of the shield will be covered in the advanced guides.

Drill 17
Starting with a strike to the right leg, followed by an cut to the left shoulder.

This is the opposite combination to Drill 15 and shows another common sequence. This is really most useful if the opponent parries the first attack with the shield. If they parry with the sword switch the second attack to their sword arm from above, with the step to the left, and when they parry that with the shield use the last part of this drill to go to the right and attack their left shoulder. Also if the opponent parries initially with the shield you can usually transfer the attack with a cut from below to the sword arm, while transferring to the other side, as shown in the second part of the drill.

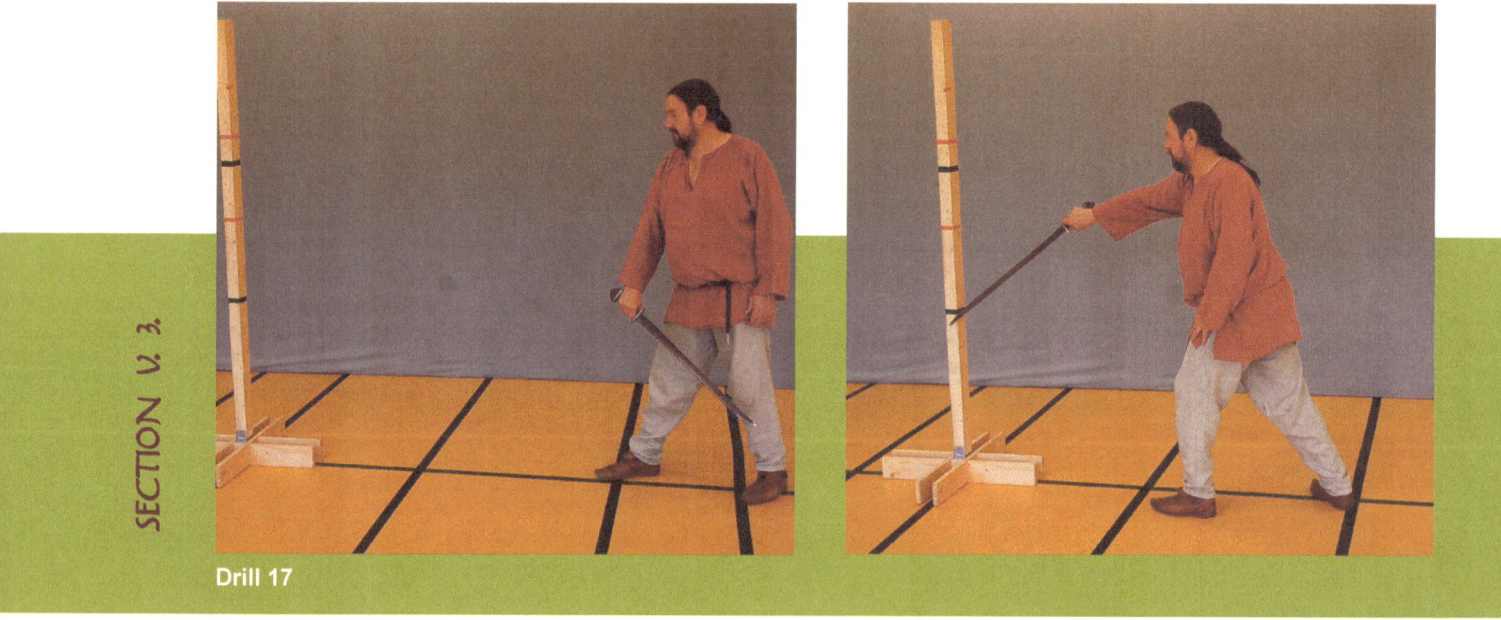

Drill 17

Start in guard position 5.

Red steps forward a full step and makes a cut from below to the opponent's right leg.

Notice that the sword cuts up into the high Ox position which withdraws the hand out of the danger zone, protects the head and prepares the sword for the next attack. This middle position could be a roof block also, stopping the opponent's counter attack before continuing on to the second half of the combination. If so the shield could then exchange into the parrying position maintaining the contact and the cover. The final step could also be a full diagonal step even further out to the right causing more problems for the opponent.

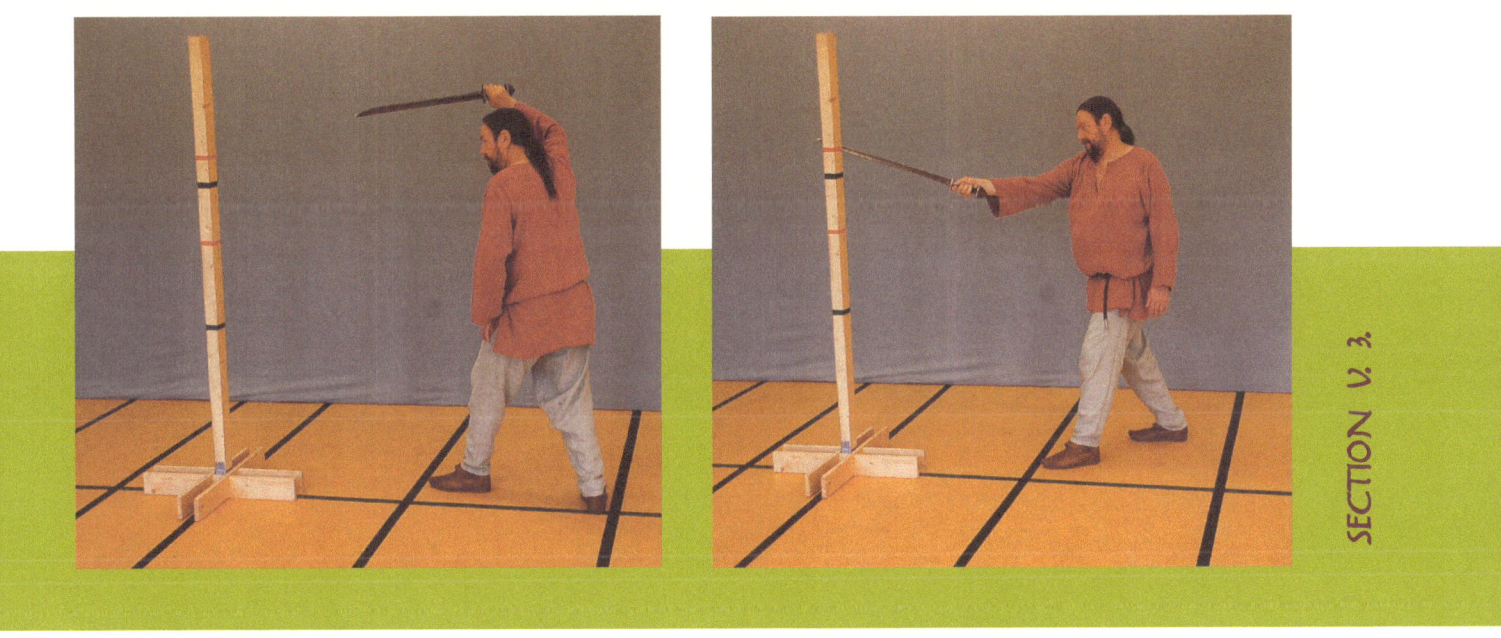

Red makes a diagonal half step to the left, this is the point Red would cover the opponent's shortest line of attack with the shield to protect against their most likely counter.

Red then finishes the sequence and cuts to the left shoulder. The fighter must be ready to switch the attack from the shoulder to a lower target if the opponent has recovered his shield back to defend.

Drill 18
Begin by striking to the left shoulder, followed by striking to the left leg.

This is a very common attacking sequence, and is designed to simply bring the shield high, and then swap to the lower target on the same side, if the opponent is slow they will be hit on the thigh. If you strike straight down from the first shield parry across the surface of their shield but without touching, this will be the quickest route. If they do not go low enough with the shield, drop below the shield rim with the sword and continue the attack from below underneath their shield by cutting upwards. If you lower your stance far enough they might be forced to ground the shield to stop your attack.

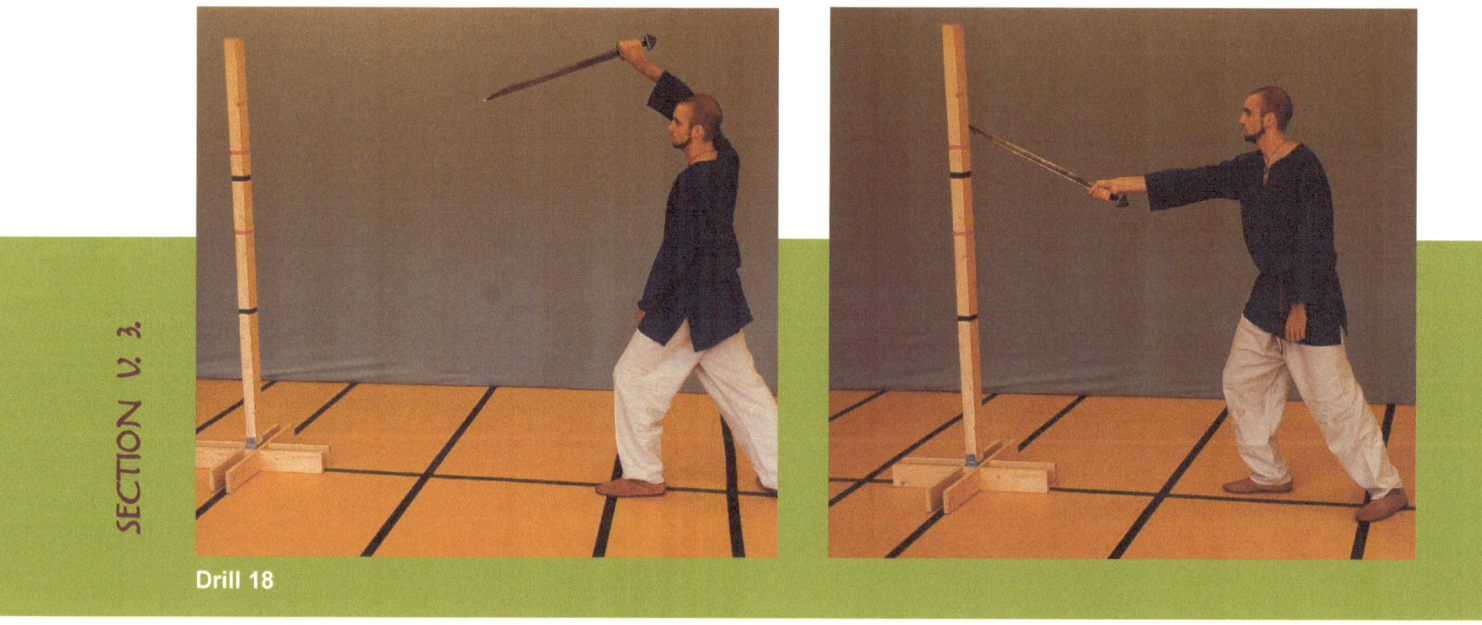

Drill 18

Blue starts in the right Ox guard position.

Blue makes a cut to the opponent's left shoulder, while stepping forward a full step.

Once again if the opponent counter attacked during the transition between attack 1 and 2, then it is possible to parry with the sword first, exchanging with the shield to facilitate the second attack. Though speed is important, timing is far more critical; dealing with a counter with a timely parry, and not being hit is much preferred over the alternative just because you are too eager to win the fight.

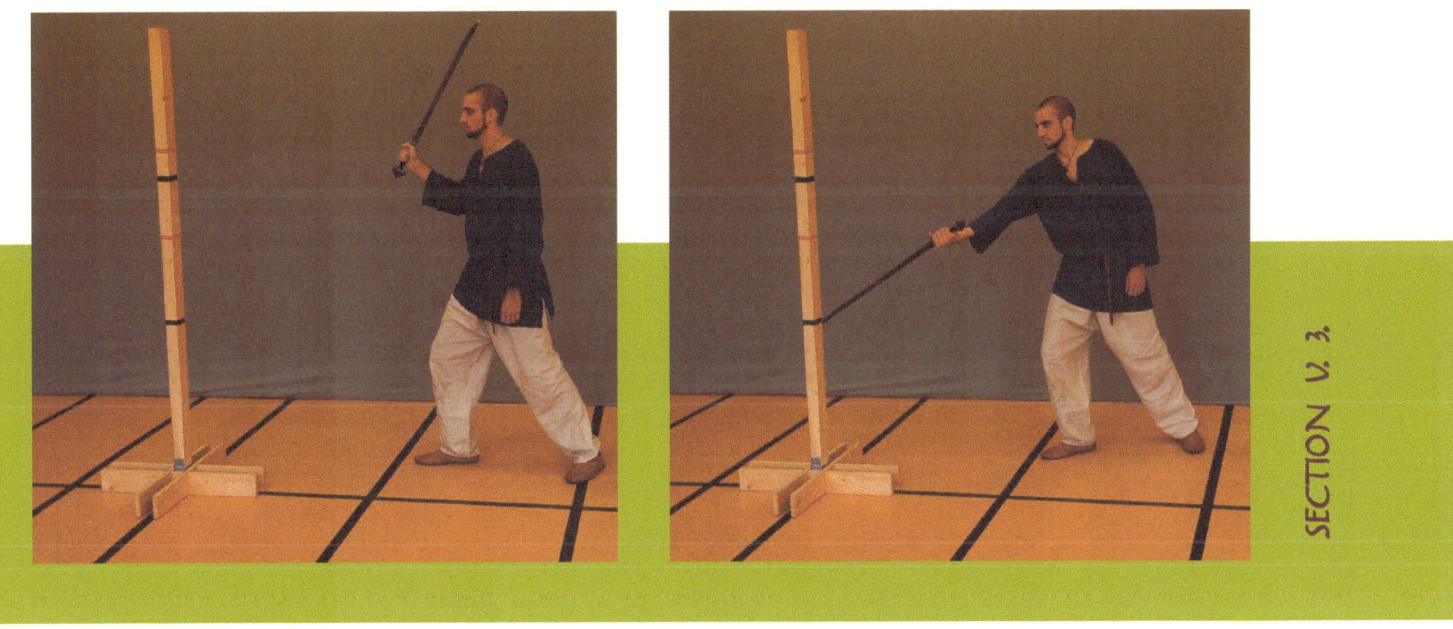

Blue moves to the right with a diagonal half step, again his shield would be positioned to protect the most likely attack from the opponent. Notice this is a move away from the weapon thereby increasing security using distance.

Finally Blue cuts to the left leg from below or above. Blue's quickest route to the leg is to drop the sword quickly down past the front face of the opponent's shield. The opponent may even loose sight of the sword, making its next appearance more of a surprise!

Drill 19
Combination Strikes with Half Step against the Pell from the Left Hander's Perspective.

This is the left hander's copy of the previous drill, the main difference is that it takes place entirely on the defenders unshielded side. Right handed people should note that this is a particularly effective tactical sequence against them. Conversely right handed people can do this same combination on the left hander's unshielded side. Both players would be advised to parry the first attack with the sword and the second with the shield.

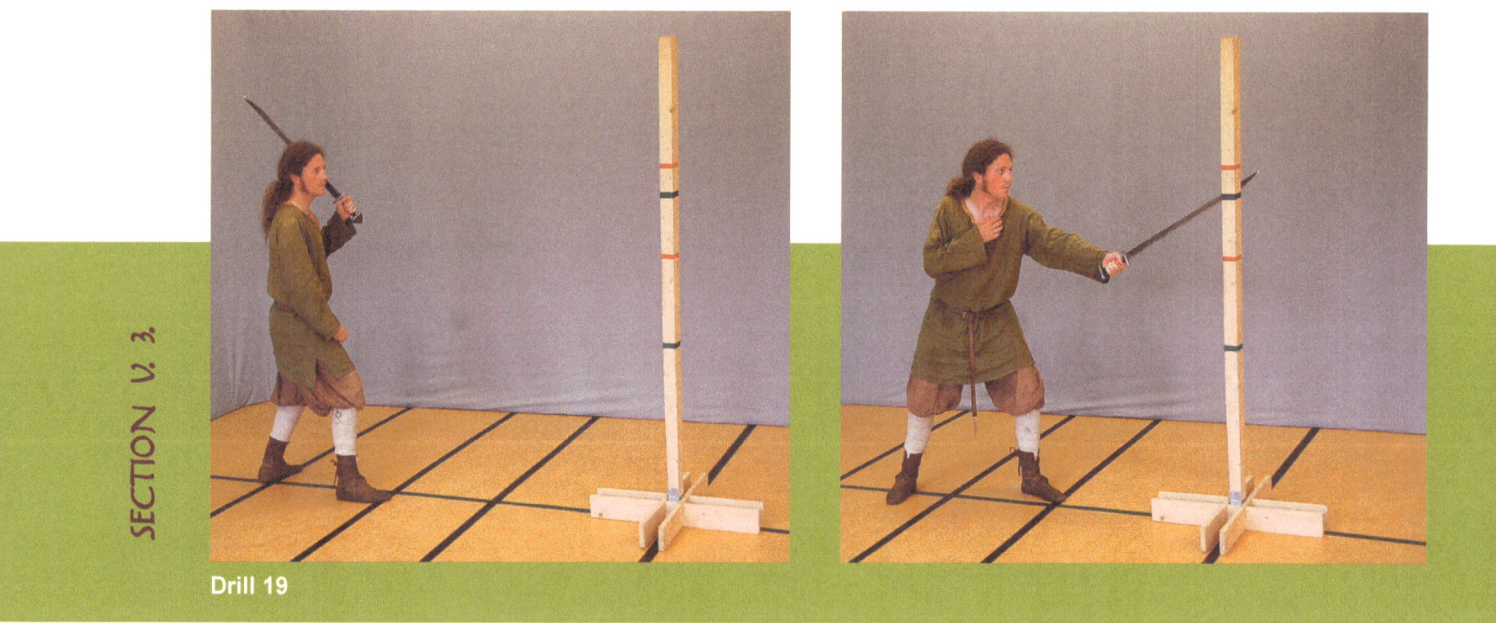

Green starts in guard position 2.

Green makes a full step forward with the left leg, and strikes to the opponent's right shoulder.

As noted previously, at this point a counter attack by the opponent is possible, and should be dealt with in the easiest way. This may mean the sword is used to parry here, after an appropriate exchange of shield for sword, the second attack in the combination can be executed. This interplay between sword and shield has to be practised and learnt, and improves with experience.

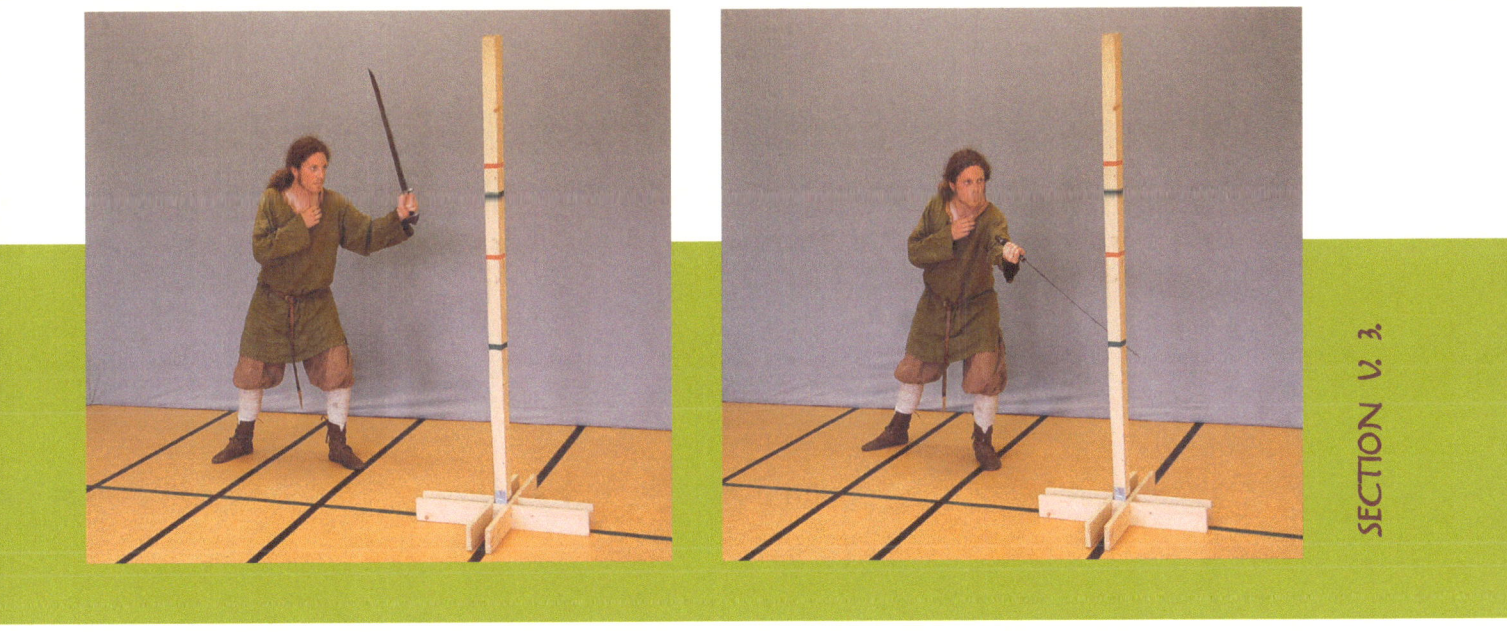

So as to move further around the unshielded side Green uses a diagonal half step to the left. Normally the shield would be positioned in the best place to deal with the opponent's sword.

Green finishes with cut from below or above against the right leg of the opponent. If this sequence was extended, it would be better to move further to the left making shield defence even more problematic. This is the nature of fights with opposite handed people, always moving to the unshielded side.

Drill 20
Initially striking to the left shoulder, followed by a strike to the right shoulder.

This is the same combination seen in Drill 9, though now using a left handed person. This is again an effective sequence because the left hander ends his move attacking the unshielded side of the opponent. If he felt that the defender was going to parry the second attack with the sword he should switch to attack the leg instead.

This is the type of initial attack which is more difficult while carrying a large shield as the sword arm can not easily be protected during this move, unless the timing of the attack is well chosen. The counter would be a parry with the shield and to attack the left handed persons' weapon arm from above or below. Some attacks should be assessed as high risk and should only be attempted when the conditions are right, though the surprise value of some attacks should not be underestimated.

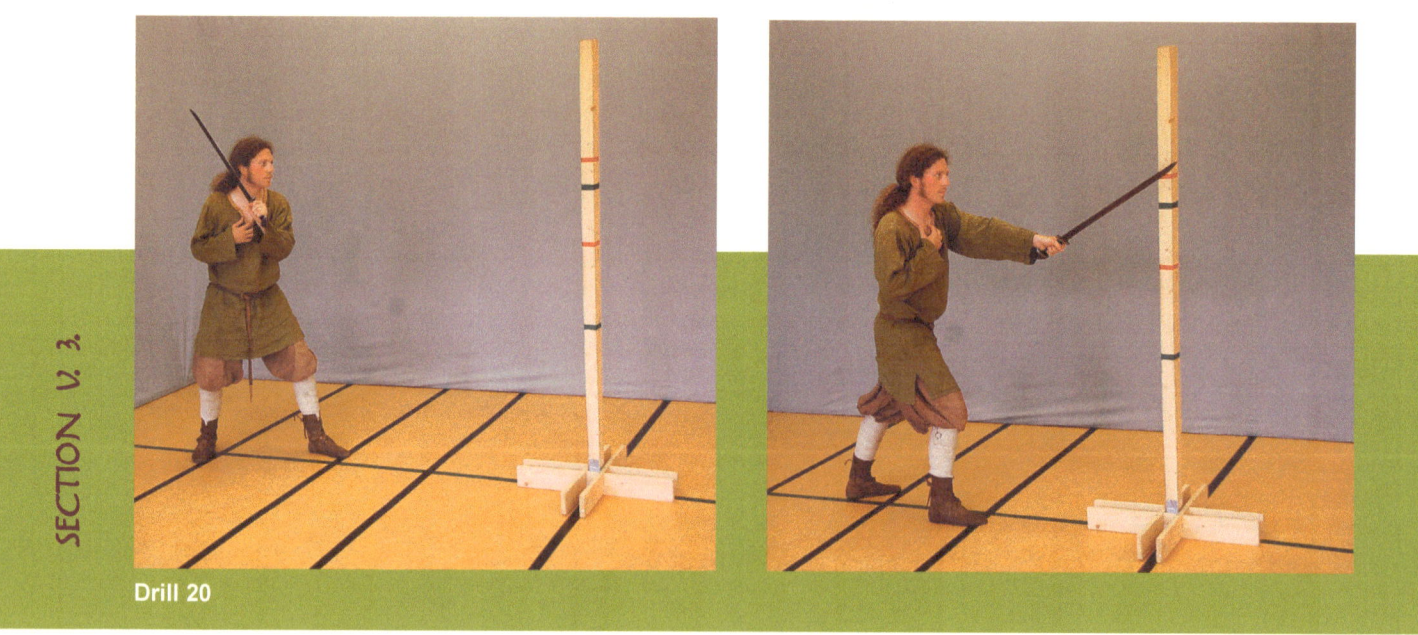

Drill 20

Green starts in guard position 3.

Green steps forward a full step with the right leg, and strikes to the opponent's left shoulder.

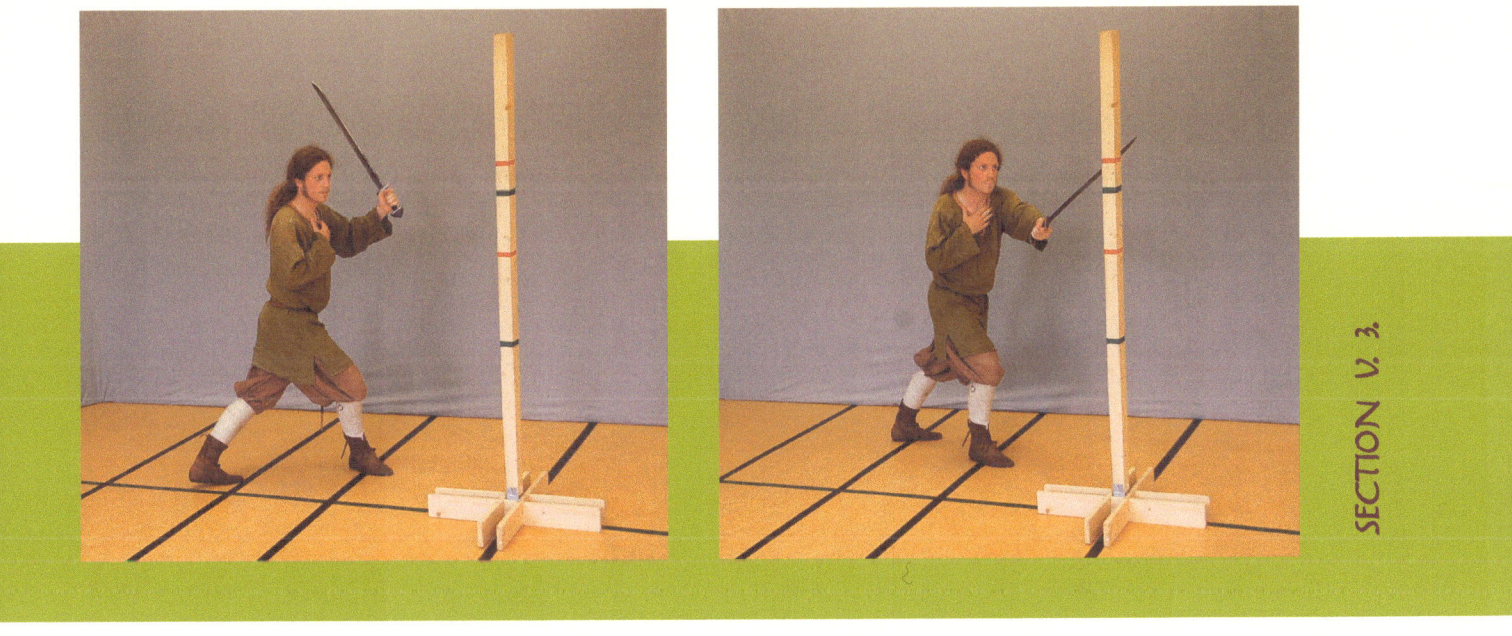

Green, moving further around the unshielded side, uses a diagonal half step to the left. The shield is positioned to deal with the opponent's sword.

Green can cut from below or above against the right shoulder of the opponent. Left handed people tend to be more at home in these positions than right handed opponents because they have more experience at fighting right hander's.

COMBINATION STRIKES WITH DIAGONAL FULL STEP AGAINST THE PELL

Drills 21-24

This is the second part of the stepping and striking combinations, first advancing towards the opponent with a half step and then stepping diagonally to the side with a full step. This form of the combination stepping drill allows the attacker to move to the side further by using the full step. This has certain advantages, not least of which is being able to reach to hit the opponent's back, even if there is a reasonable cover from the shield. This type of stepping really comes into its own when we study feints, especially if the opponent is too slow to respond to the change of angle. So this section is extremely important to understand completely, and to practice as much as possible, with or without a partner. The initial half step sets up threat that the opponent must react to or they may be hit, this reaction indicates to the attacker what the next stage will be in the sequence. The attacker must remain flexible, so that they can switch the attack to the openings as they appear, while moving to the correct position. The attacker must also be aware of the counter attacks and counter moves of the opponent during his switch of position. We will discuss these variations more in more advanced guides.

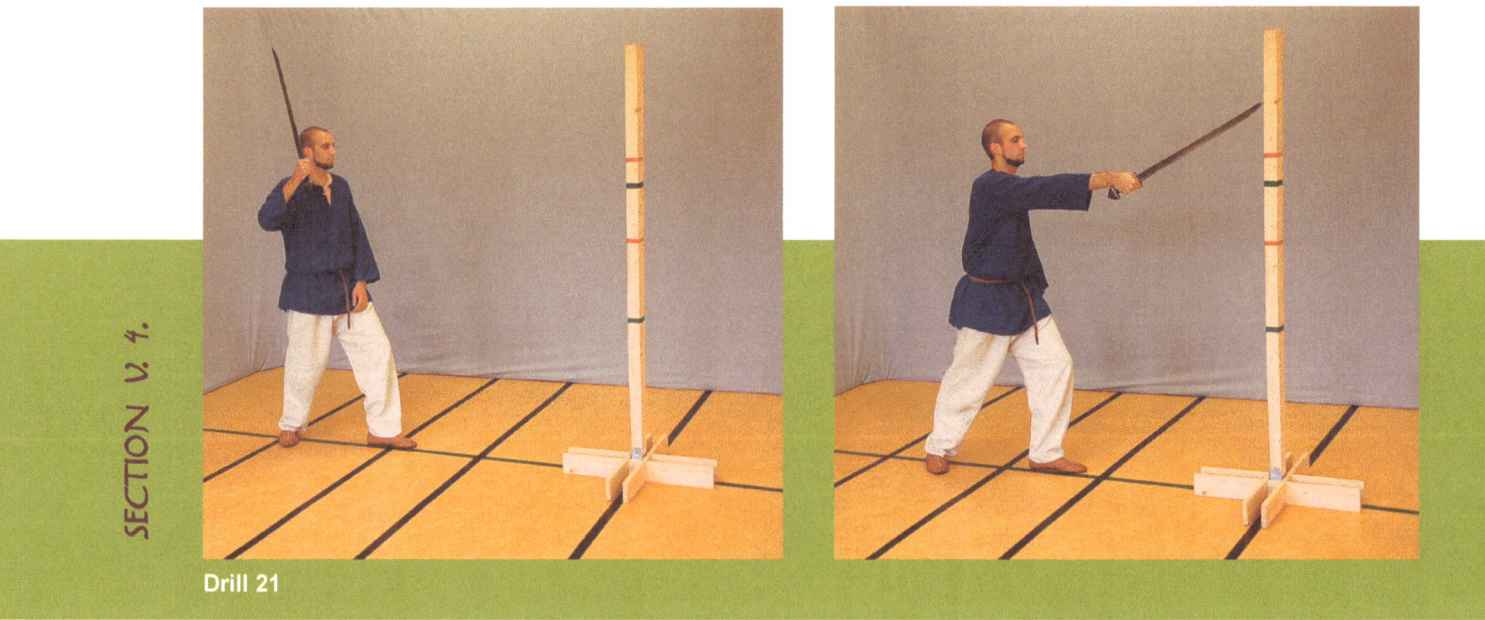

Drill 21

Blue starts in guard position 1 or position 2.

Blue uses a half step and strikes to the head,

Drill 21
Begin by striking to the head with a half step, followed by a strike to the opponent's left leg while using a full step.

This is a fairly typical sequence, using a high attack to move the opponent's shield away from defending a larger target and then swapping to that target. The strike to the left leg could be from above or below. You should have moved sufficiently far away from the opponent's weapon arm to be out of his range.

The shield should cover the high line if the opponent's sword is above the shoulder, and could be more in the centre if below the shoulder.

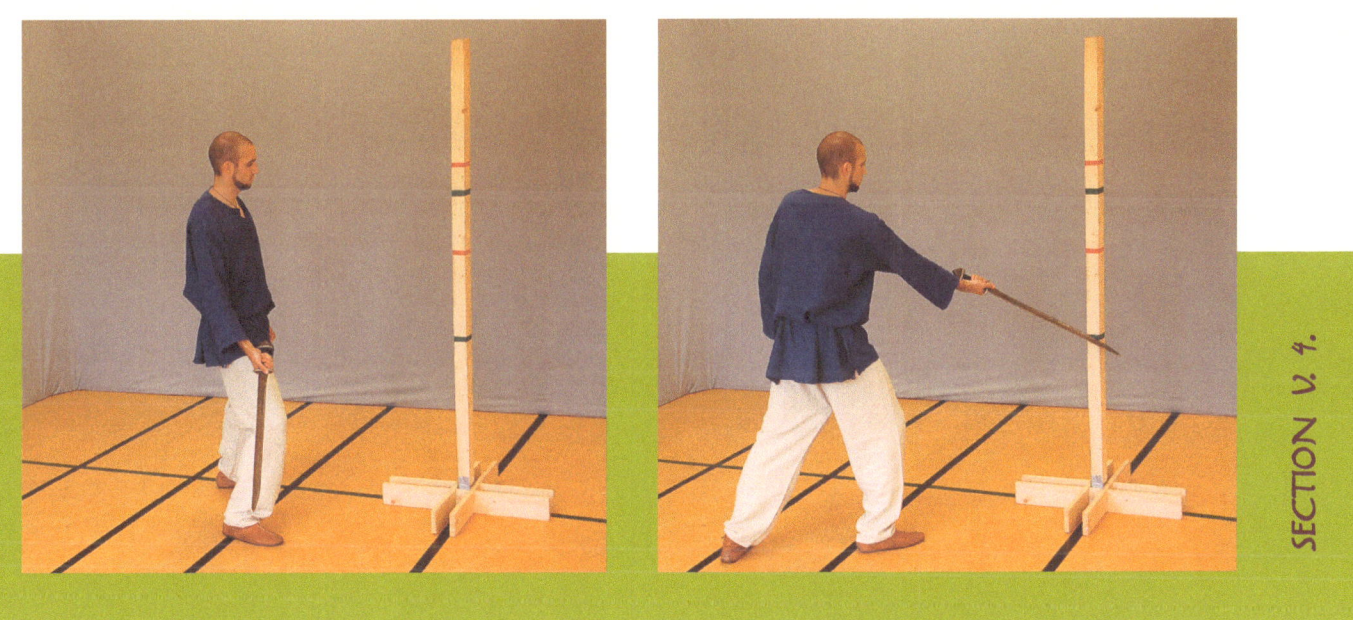

Using a diagonal full step to the right, Blue moves away from the opponent's sword and increases his reach on the opponent's shielded side.

Blue uses this advantage to cut from above or below against the left leg. If the opponent's shield has recovered position, by lowering his stance by bending the knees, Blue can slip the sword under the lower rim of the opponent's shield to cut up behind it. This movement will be covered in the advanced guides.

Drill 22
This starts by striking to the right shoulder with a half step, and continues with striking to the leg on the same side with a full step.

This is one of the best combinations we can make if the opponent allows us to get to the flank without turning to meet the manoeuvre, as the whole unshielded side is open. The diagonal step to the side can really open up the targets, and if the opponent tries to parry only using the sword he can be in great danger of being hit. Also if he parries the first or second attack with the sword you could exchange your shield for your sword and start with a new combination!

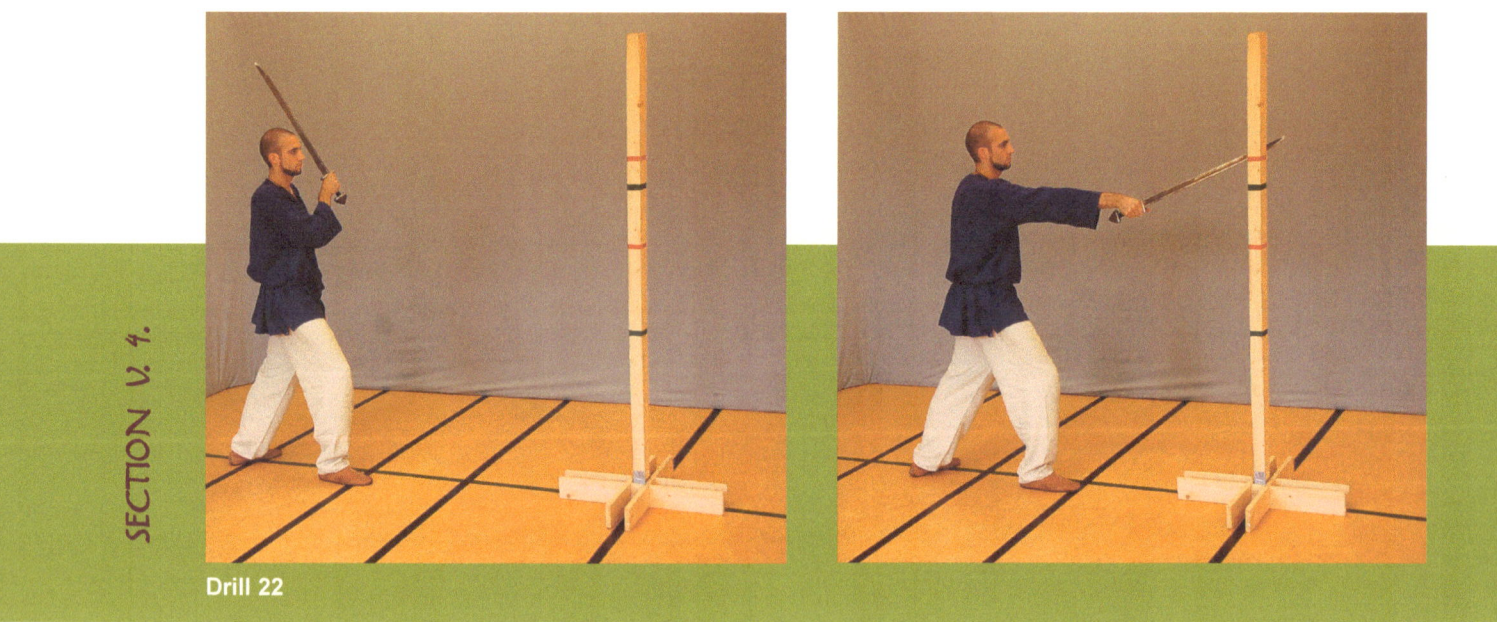

Drill 22

Starts in guard position 3 with the right leg forward.

After the normal half step forward Blue strikes to the right shoulder.

During the transition to the second attack the shield must work in close proximity to the sword, covering the attacking lines of the opponent. The sword blade in this case usually must travel across the face of the fighter's own shield to reach the target. It is essential to practice all these drills with a shield after learning the sequences.

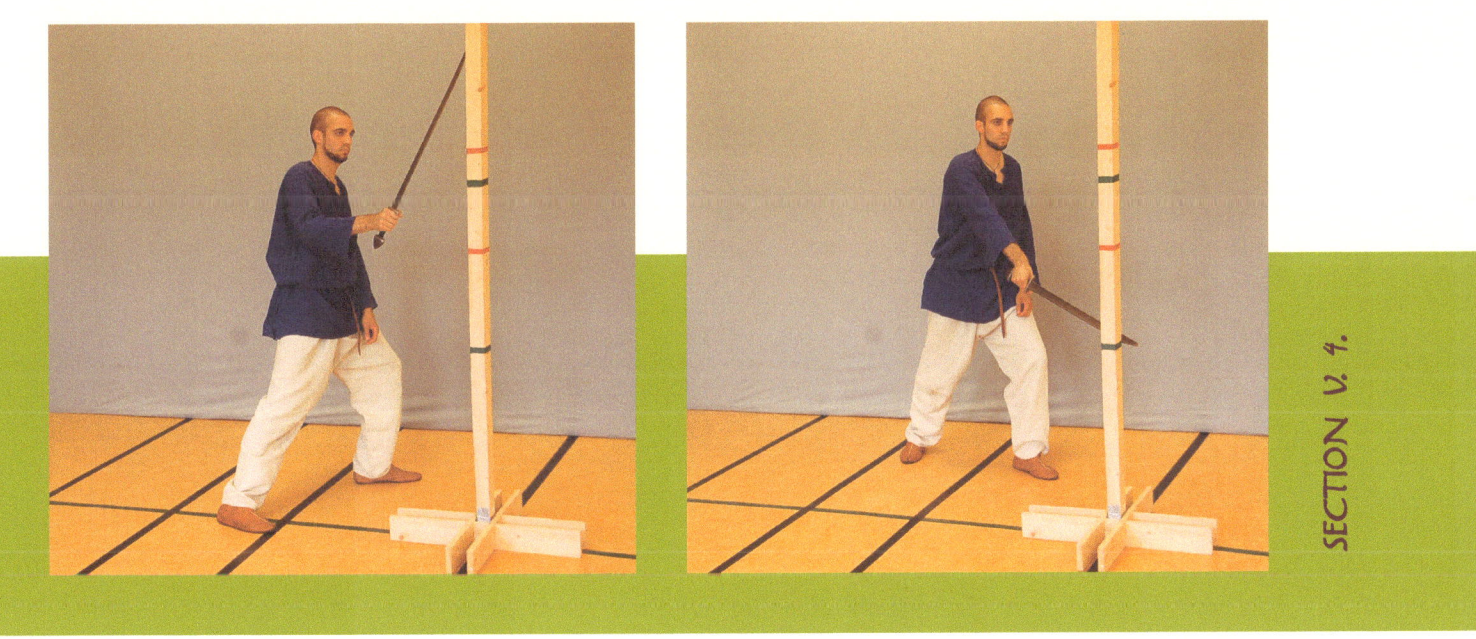

Blue completes the movement using a diagonal full step to the left.

Blue cuts to the right leg from above. If the opponent has stepped back with the right leg, the left leg may still be open and can be targeted.

Drill 23
The first strike is to the left thigh with a half step, followed by striking to the left shoulder with a full step.

This sequence exploits excessive movement of the shield by attacking low to the leg and then switching to the shoulder on the same side, a theme we have shown several times. With the wide step out to the side this opens up more of the opponent to be hit. Further guides will show other ways of exploiting this situation against even large shields.

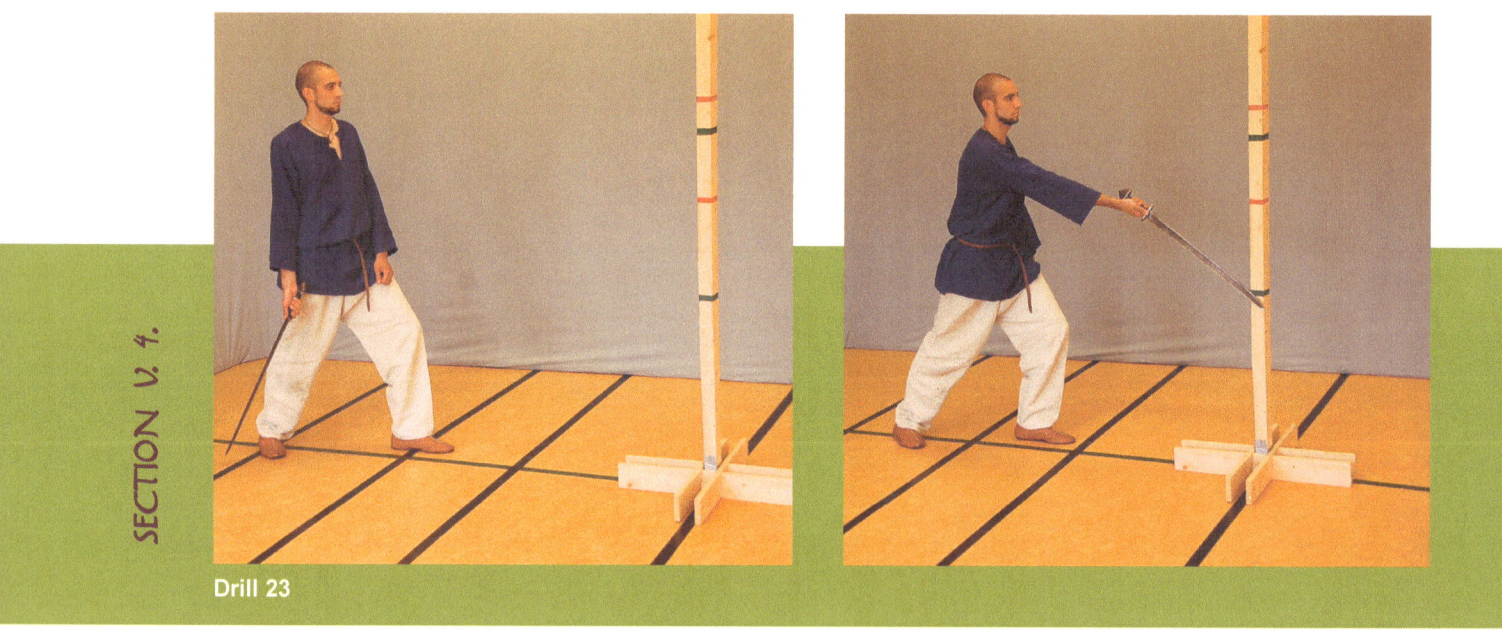

Drill 23

Blue starts in guard position 4.

Blue initialises the threat by making a half step forward while cutting from below to the left leg. This should obtain a reaction from the opponent, setting him up for the next cut.

Take note that the middle picture where we show the transition to the next cut is always shown as a full pull back to cut again. When the fighter has learnt to generate power within a smaller movement, this large movement is not necessary and will be much quicker. To refine movements to be more efficient takes time and experience and it is best to start with the complete movement and work towards smaller.

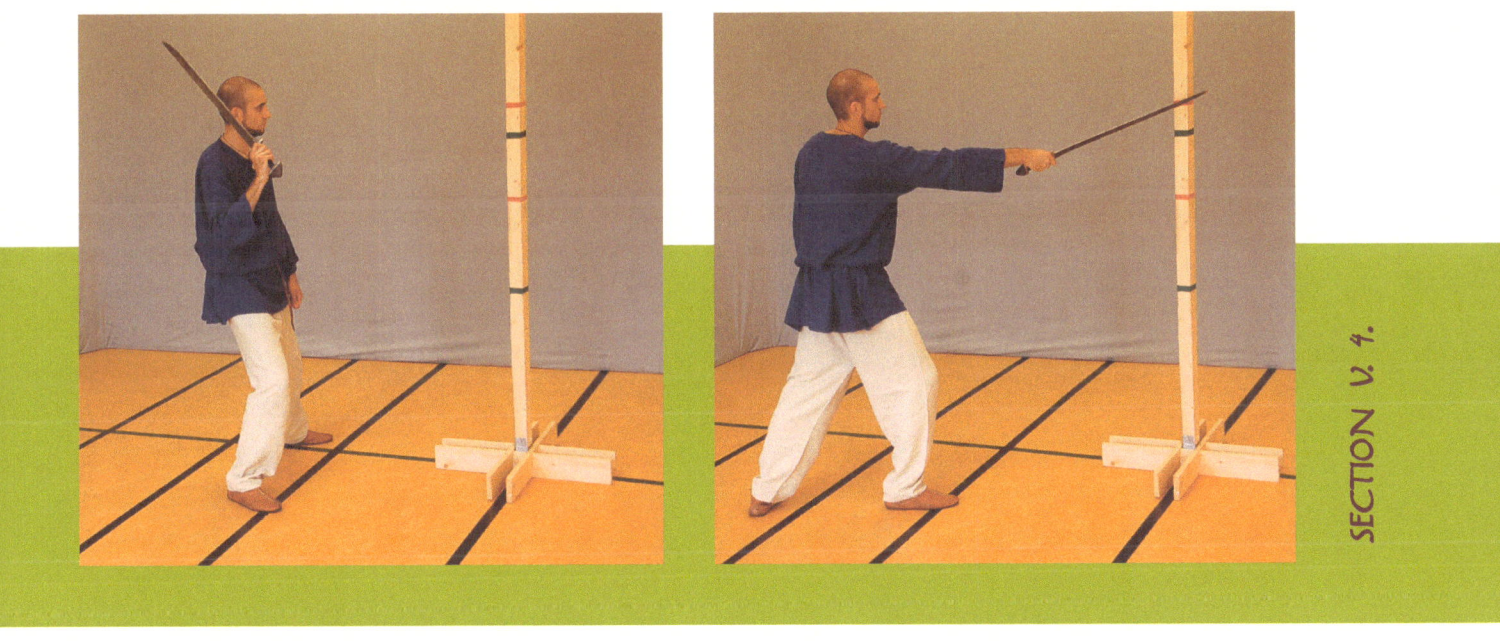

Blue continues with a diagonal half step to the right. This increases the pressure and moves away from the opponent's weapon, thereby increasing the security.

At the same time cutting to the left shoulder or arm. The shield should be positioned to protect the sword arm, unless the proximity of the opponent's weapon warrants another placement.

Drill 24
After striking to the right thigh with a half step, the second strike is to the right shoulder full step.

This is the same manoeuvre as Drill 22 though with targets reversed, going high to low. With this diagonal step you open up the unshielded side again, and allow the possibility exchanging sword for shield. Be sure to cover your movement with your own shield whenever you cross in front of the opponent. Do not be caught out with a lazy shield after you have closed the distance. The sword and shield coordination must be thought through slowly. This is a tricky movement which requires training and good timing, not least with the shield. The final attack could be a cut from below as required.

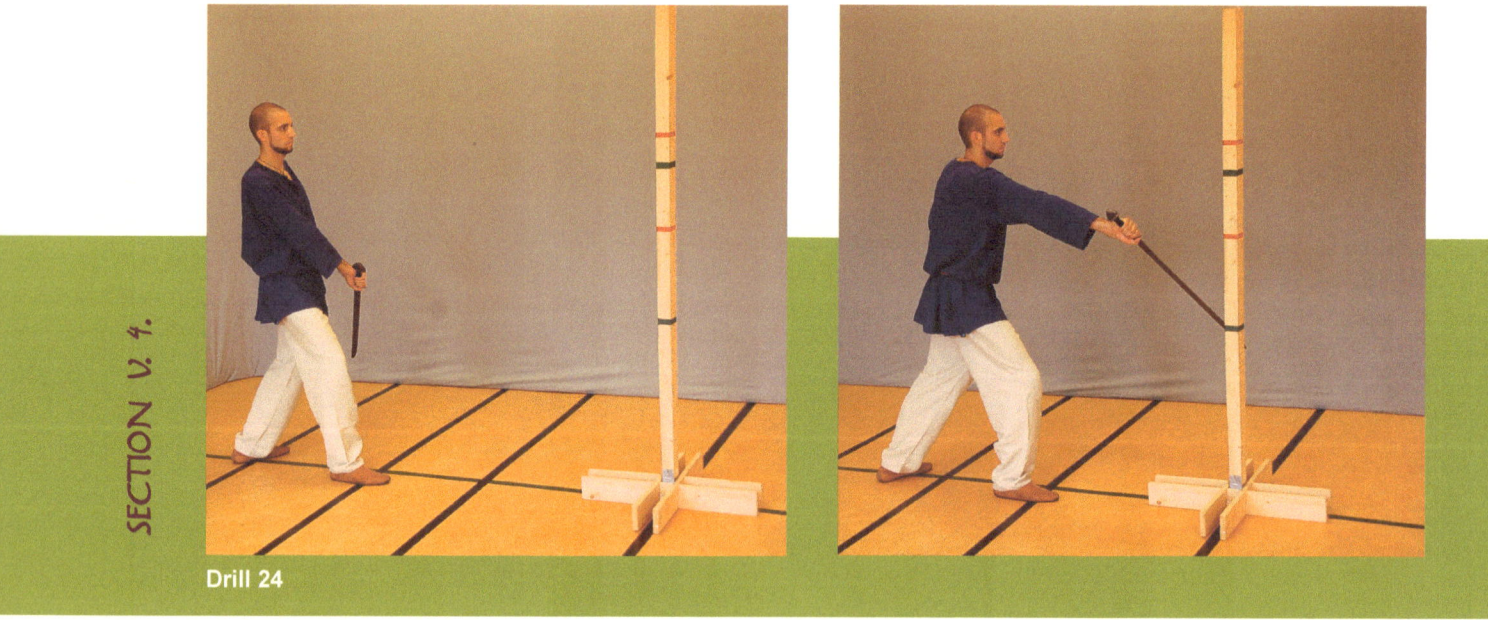

Drill 24

Blue starts in guard position 5 with the right leg forward.

Blue starts the sequence with a cut from below to the opponent's right leg, while stepping forward a half step. The sword arm is exposed, and should be protected by the shield.

The final attack could be changed to a low attack to the leg by simply turning the wrist over, or cutting down onto the leg from the transition position.

The way that the final attack avoids the opponent's sword and shield even when in close proximity of the target is sometimes just a matter of blade angle. This angle adjustment can be quite small, just enough to find a small hole in the defence, though critical if the blow is to land. This a difficult adjustment to show in pictures and usually comes through experience.

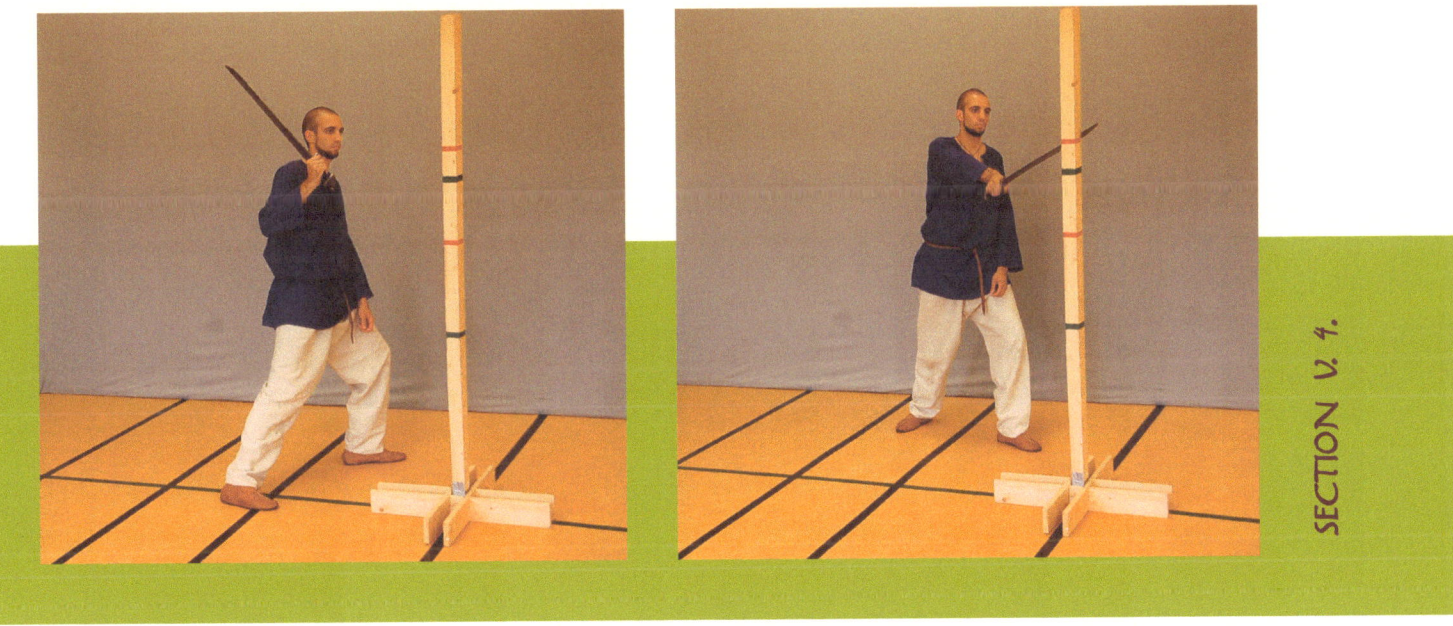

Blue steps to the left, bringing the sword into position to strike at the next target.

Blue finishes the sequence with a cut from above to the right shoulder or arm. This cut could also be from below against the same target. Cutting from below may be easier or safer if the shield used is large.

SECTION VI – PARTNER DRILLS

COMBINATION STRIKES WITH DIAGONAL STEPPING

Drills 1-10

In each drill the first attack will be executed using a half step straight forward, followed by a diagonal step to the side using a full step.

Combining attacks with offline footwork is so important that we admonish the student to study this aspect in great depth. This is also the essence of feints, where attacks are not completed but changed to another target while the initial movement draws away the defence. This form of combat has many advantages, not the least of which is to be able to confuse inexperienced fighters leading to a quick hit. There are several down sides to feinting, and usually experienced fighters are ready for them with counter moves of their own. We do not explore feinting in the Beginners Guides because they are best learned after combination strikes, as they are essentially the same though with a different emphasis on cut path and target, and the idea of only making one motion with the sword.

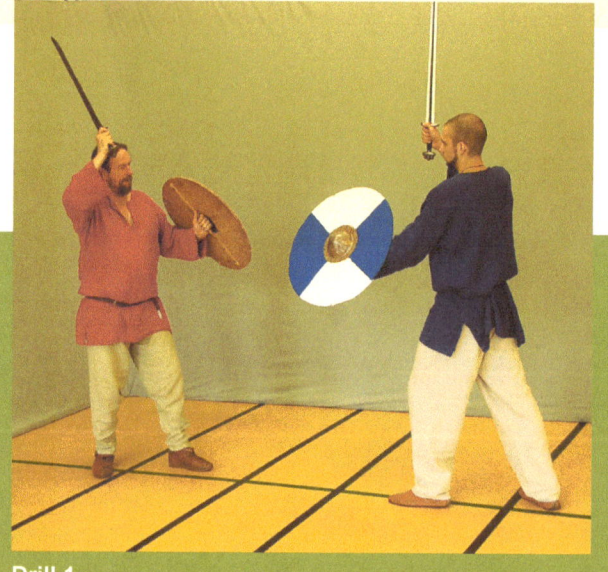

Drill 1

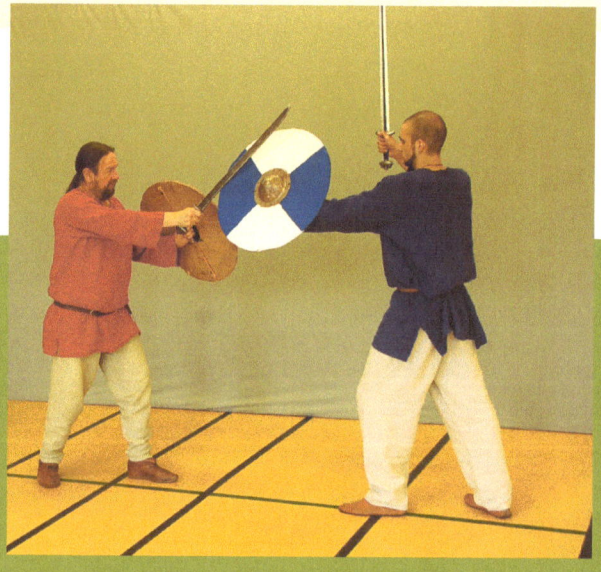

Both start in guard position 1.

Red attacks the head making a half step forward. Blue steps a half step back and parries with the shield.

Drill 1
Beginning with an attack to the left shoulder, followed by a striking to the left leg from above or below.

We have seen this simple sequence several times from different sides. The attacker wishes to exploit movement of the shield, while angling off to the side to increase the number of targets. There are numerous minor variations in this technique, including step width and angle, and where and how the sword moves to the target; such as moving the sword down over the face of the shield after the parry.

Because of the necessity to show a sequence that the student can learn from, the opponent in these pictures always seems to stop reacting to the second attack. Sometimes, it has been noted, that in a real fight people freeze in place and make no movement or very little. This can also happen in sparring, though mostly opponents do something, in this case just flow seamlessly into another sequence and keep the initiative. This is the real art of the fight, to keep applying technique until one is successful, while making sure you are not hit in return.

Note that Red's shield is positioned to take care of high line attacks to the shoulder and head. The distance created by diagonal stepping automatically protects the low line.

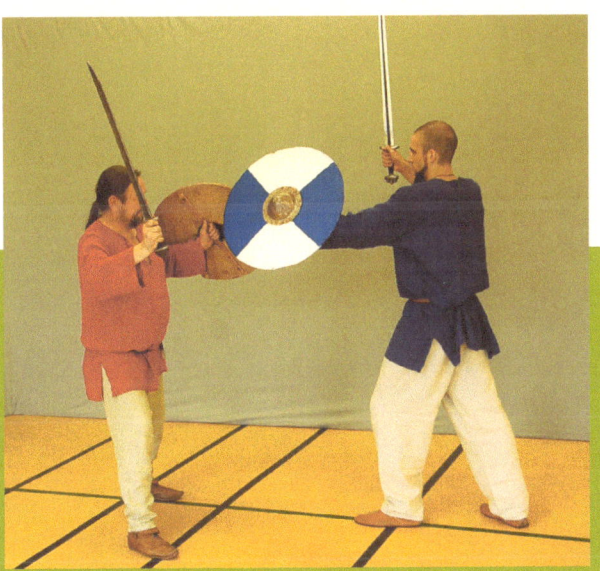

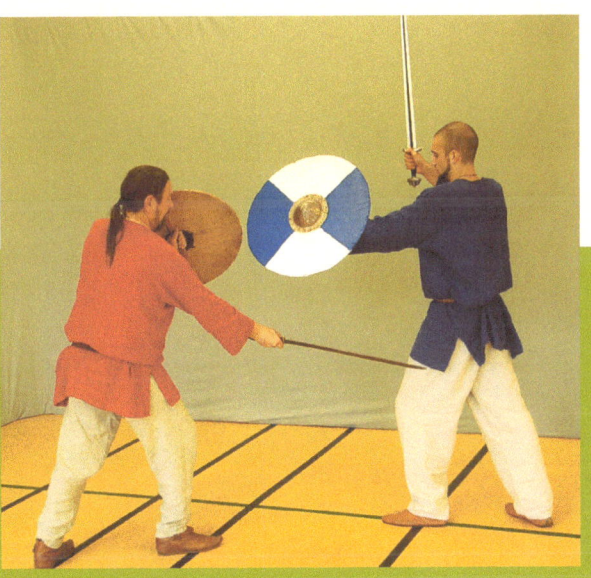

Red makes a full step to diagonally to the right, angling away from the sword of the opponent. Keeping distance is extremely important!

Red attacks Blue's left leg from above.

Drill 2
The first attack is to the right shoulder, the second is to the leg on the same side.

This is almost a repeat of the previous drill though with an initial attack to the shoulder, if you are not using a full body target this is the preferred method. Also it is more likely that they will defend with the shield in this position, whereas if you attack the head we recommend that people defend with the sword so that you do not loose sight of the opponent. It is sometimes better for the attacker if the opponent commits his shield rather than the sword.

Note that the difference is the end attack is from below not above, this is preferred if the opponent manages to recover the shield back to defend. Drop the stance as you strike and come under the shield with the attack. This sometimes requires you to flip the blade under the lower edge of the shield to position the sword behind the shield. The opponent then as very little chance of recovery from this position.

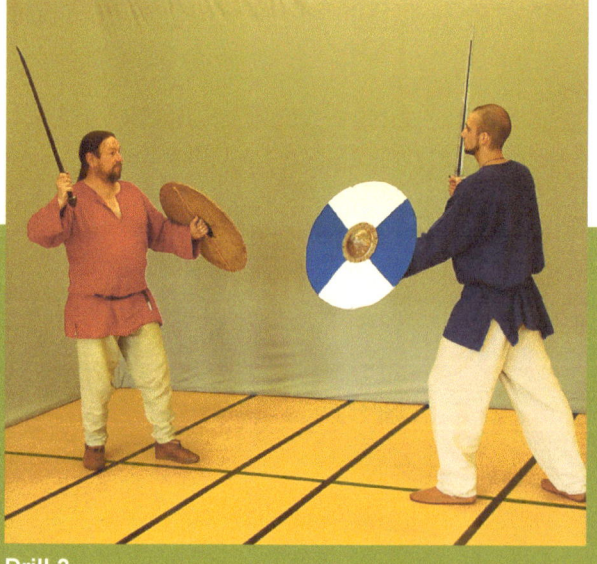

Drill 2

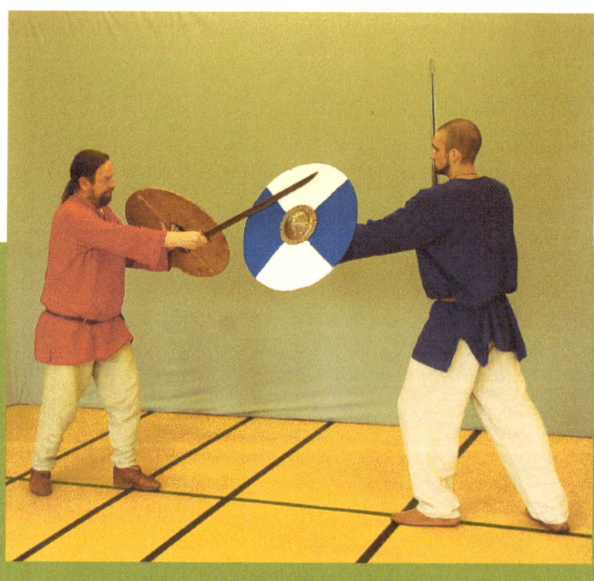

Both start in guard position 2

Red attacks the left shoulder making a half step forward. Blue steps a half step back and parries with the shield.

The static nature of the defender is not a problem at this stage as this is a training sequence. The object of practice is to program the muscle memory so that the movements can be repeated under stress. Once the defender can move in any direction, the level of complication of the situation increases dramatically. Therefore the chance of learning the sequence from a book is greatly reduced.

More complex situations will be dealt with in later books though the object on any sequence is to teach a principle. These principles can be then applied to any situation encountered later. Techniques learnt in this book should be seen as stepping stones, several strung together will, if correctly applied, lead to advantageous situations. One technique should flow seamlessly into the next so that the opponent has no chance to recover from the initial surprise.

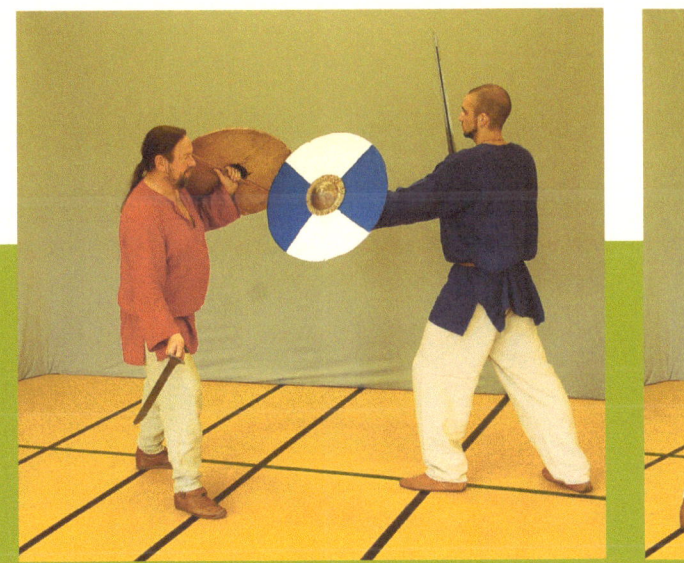

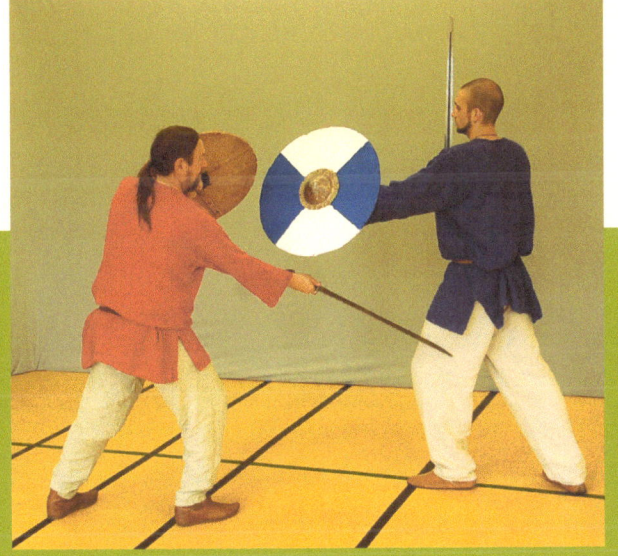

Red makes a full step diagonally to the right, positioning the sword for the attack.

Red attacks Blue's left leg from below. This could also be a thrust into the side, we cover that in book 3. This is a sequence that will occur thousands of times in the course of training, and knowing all the ways to exploit the situation will bring many rewards.

Drill 3
Beginning with a strike to the right shoulder, followed by an attack to the leg on the same side.

The aim here is again to move out to the unshielded side of the opponent, by engaging their sword and closing the distance in complete safety. Once the opponent's sword is occupied, you cover the line of their sword to your body with your shield and then disengage swords, while swapping to the new target; the right leg.

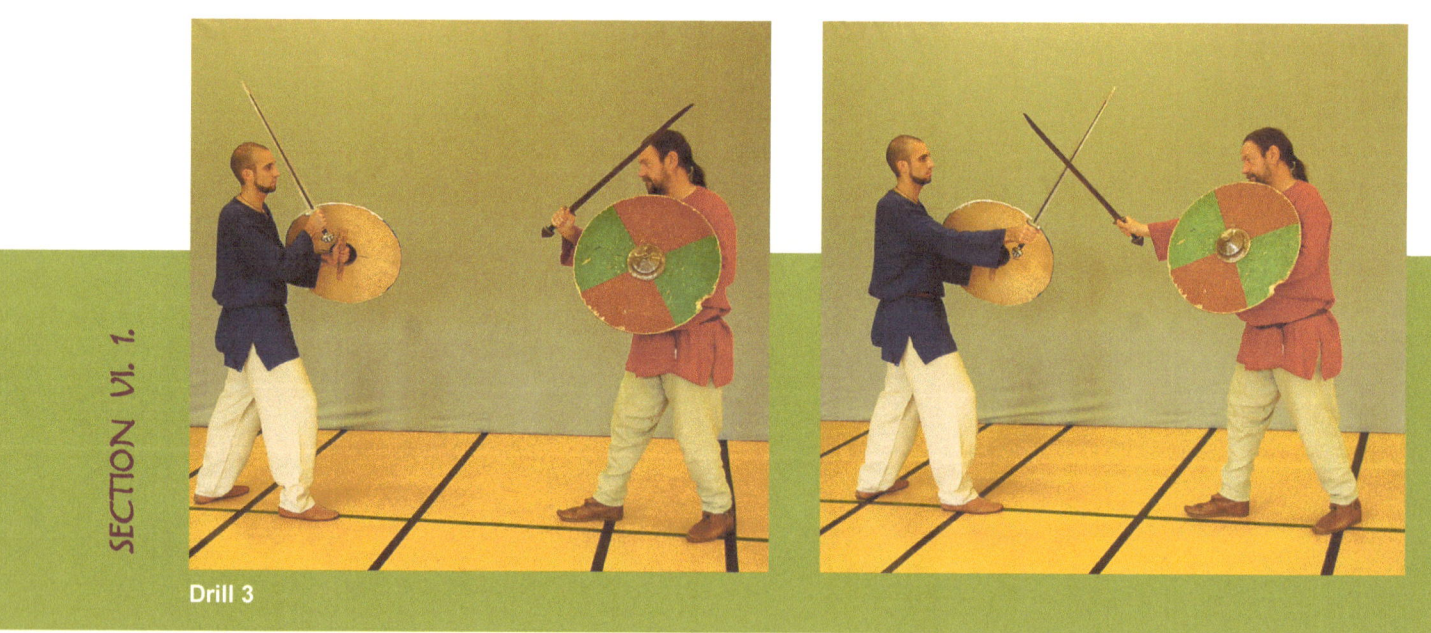

Drill 3

Both start in guard position 3.

Red attacks the right shoulder making a half step forward. Blue steps a half step back and parries with the sword.

This sequence is also excellent if you can exchange the sword for the shield on the outside especially if you can control the opponent's sword hand with the edge of the shield. In this case if they just drop the sword down and make parry 4, you can still engage the sword hand with the edge of the shield and hit. These subtle application of technique beyond what you have been taught makes all the difference in a fight. The realisation that techniques do not stop until the opponent is overwhelmed is a key element in being a successful fighter. If you can continuously string combinations together in a manner which maintains the initiative, you will have make a great leap forward in development.

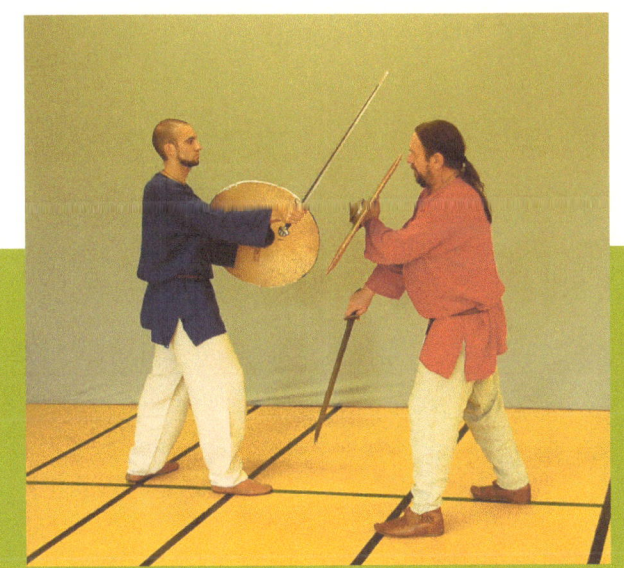

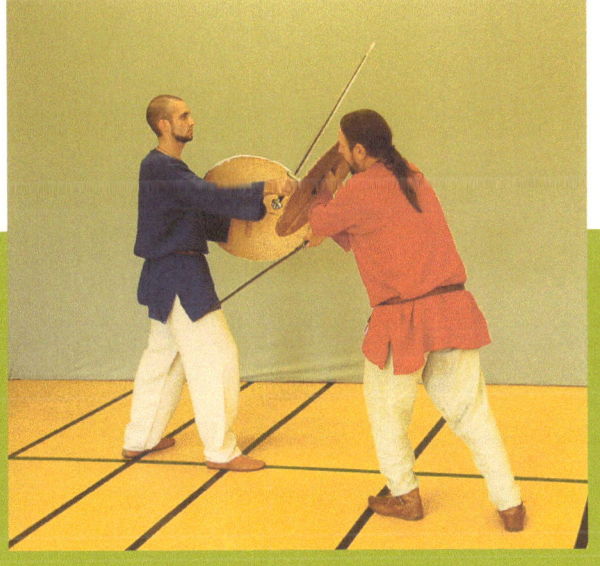

Red makes a full step to diagonally to the left, while preparing the sword for the next attack and also placing the shield to cover the expected counter attacks of the opponent.

Red then attacks Blue's right leg from below. Red could exchange shield for sword making Blue's job even harder. Even if Blue manages to drop the sword down to parry the attack, Red could immediately strike to the upper arm point downward, continuing the attacking sequence.

Drill 4
Initially attacking the left leg, continuing with a strike to the shoulder on the same side.

All combination drills have in common a similar theme, force the opponent to parry in one area, which in turn opens up another area that you can reach quickly. With diagonal full steps even large shields can be defeated in this way. Here this is again all on one side of the body, and on the opponent's shield side, the diagonal movement succeeds in also moving away from their weapon.

We will explore how knowledge of blade and shield geometry can be used to defeat a good defence in the advanced guides.

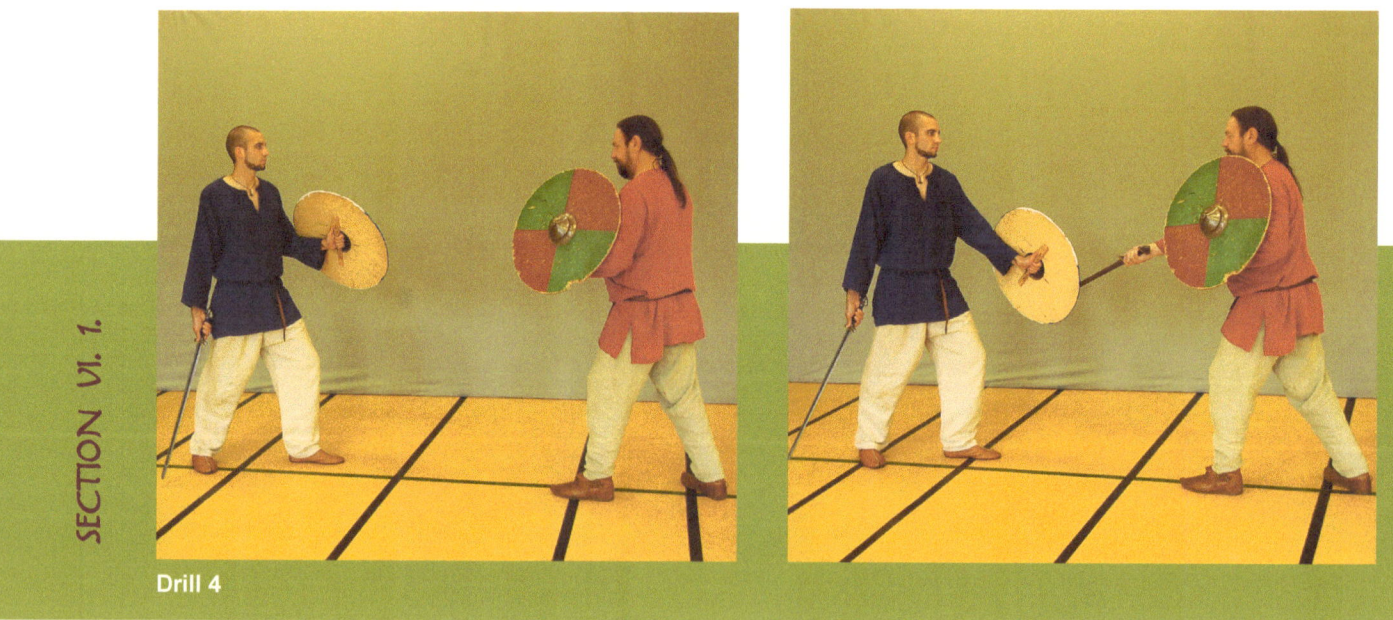

Drill 4

Both start in guard position 4.

Red attacks the left leg from below making a half step forward. Blue steps a half step back and parries with the shield.

Here is another example of multiple opportunities. Blue may recover the shield back to parry this second shoulder attack. As you see this happening alter the attack back down to the leg while stepping forward another half step. As can be seen in the last picture there is also some shield contact, this is also important, as this give you information about where the opponent's shield is and if it moves.

The subject of shield position and contact is complex and we cover some of the aspects in the advanced guides. Suffice to say that if the opponent moves his shield back to parry, you could, if not threatened press on the edge of the shield making it swivel, opening up the target again.

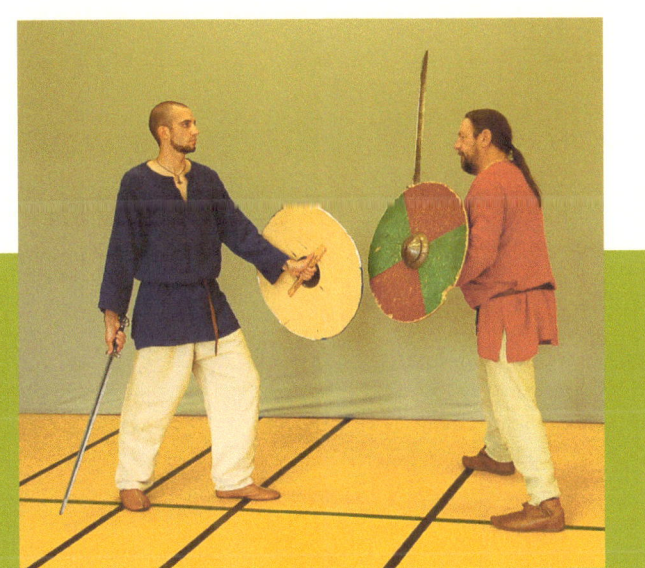
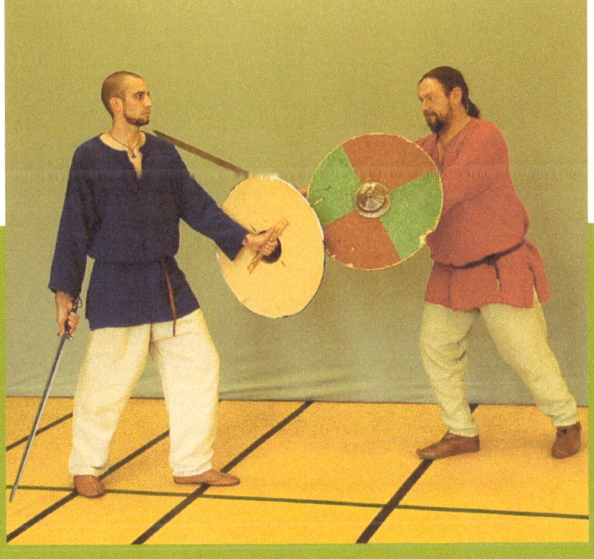

Red makes a full step to diagonally to the right, repositioning the sword and interposing the shield to cover expected attacks of Blue.

Finally Red attacks Blue's left shoulder from above. If the opponent had a large shield in this position then Red would have attacked the head, almost forcing a raised shield, which naturally could be exploited by cutting next below the shield to the leg.

Drill 5
Starting with a strike to the right leg; followed by an attack to the shoulder on the same side.

On the unshielded side of the opponent we can repeat the same theme, with the added advantage of off siding their shield. If they parry with the sword this will interfere with the proper use of the shield, if they use their shield it will be drawn well out of position. If their shield is out of position you can then switch sides and exploit that situation as their sword will almost certainly be masked by the shield, making the transfer to the other side safer.

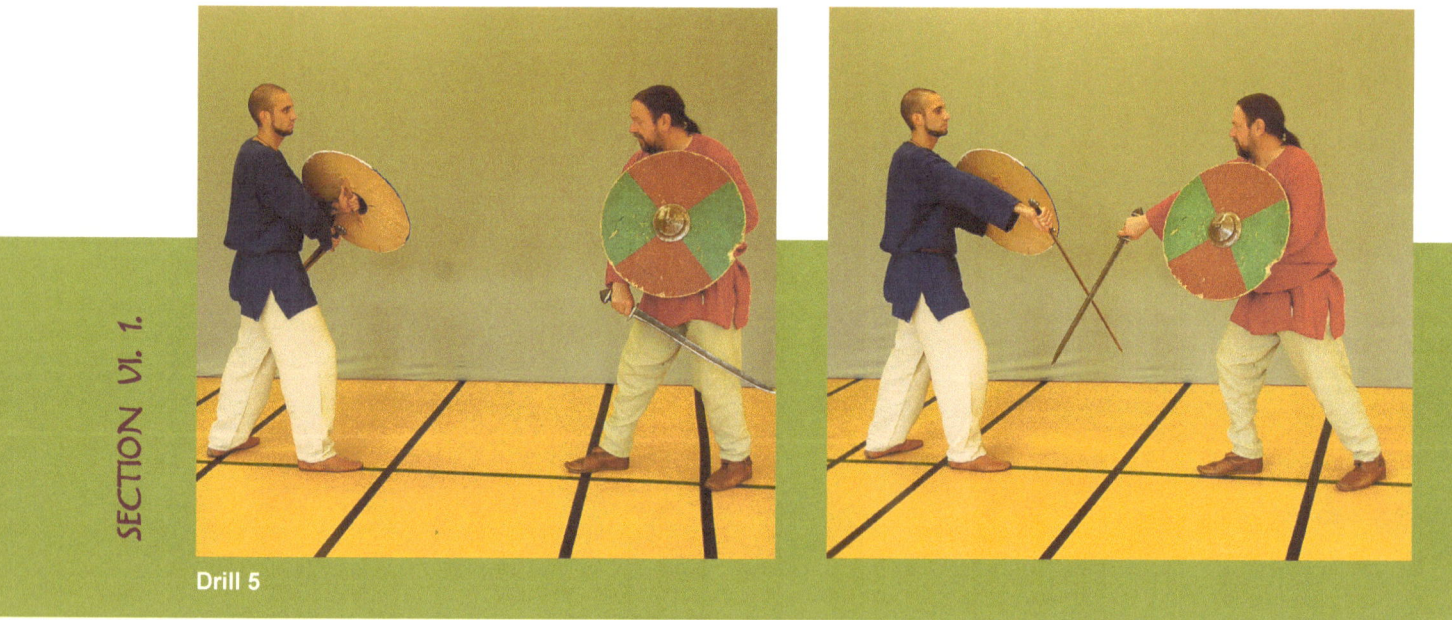

Drill 5

Both start in guard position 5.

Red attacks the right leg from below, making a half step forward. Blue steps a half step back and parries with the sword.

Even if the opponent parries the second attack with the sword you can switch the attack to the right leg from above, thus the tactical sequence continues.

This is another example of using a middle tempo to change line. This means that, had the opponent utilised a sword parry against the last attack shown in this drill, as he is in the process of making it, you change your attacking line to hit the leg. This is an advanced concept, the use of a middle tempo, but a concept than nevertheless needs an introduction some time in the student's development. This, once understood, is a real advantage and it was exploited to the full by the masters of old.

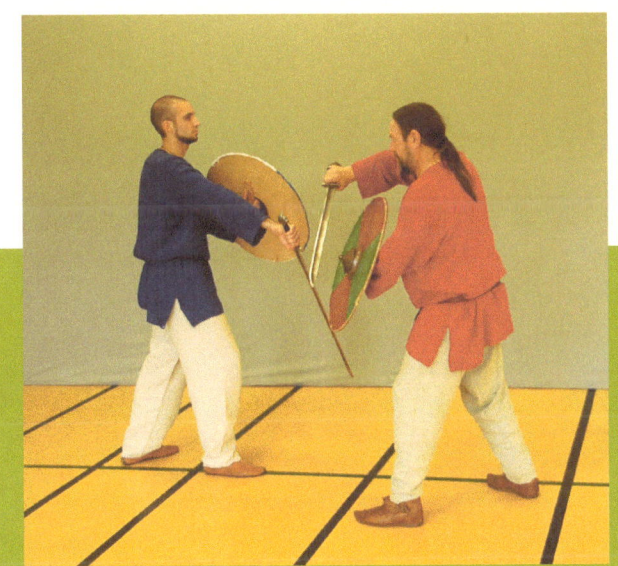

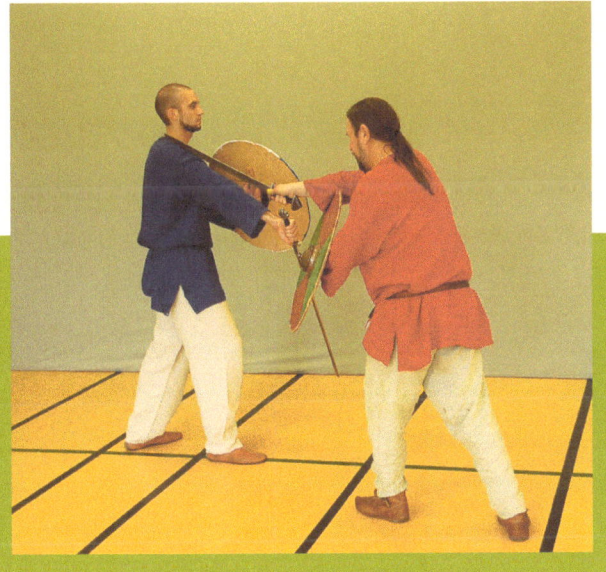

Red makes a full step to diagonally to the left, preparing both the sword and shield for the next part. Both cover the expected attacks of the opponent's sword while the step is taking place.

Then Red attacks Blue's right shoulder from above.

DISARMS
Drill 6-9

Drill 6
Pommel grab against a right handed person by a right handed person.

Disarming is not often seen though when someone is successful with this technique it looks spectacular and often leaves the opponent confused. The move is possible with the sword point up as in this example or with it down. You can see that the left hand goes over the right in the pictures, though in the case of the sword point being in the down position, such as in a roof parry, the hand would go underneath the sword arm to reach the pommel. These moves must be well practiced to succeed.

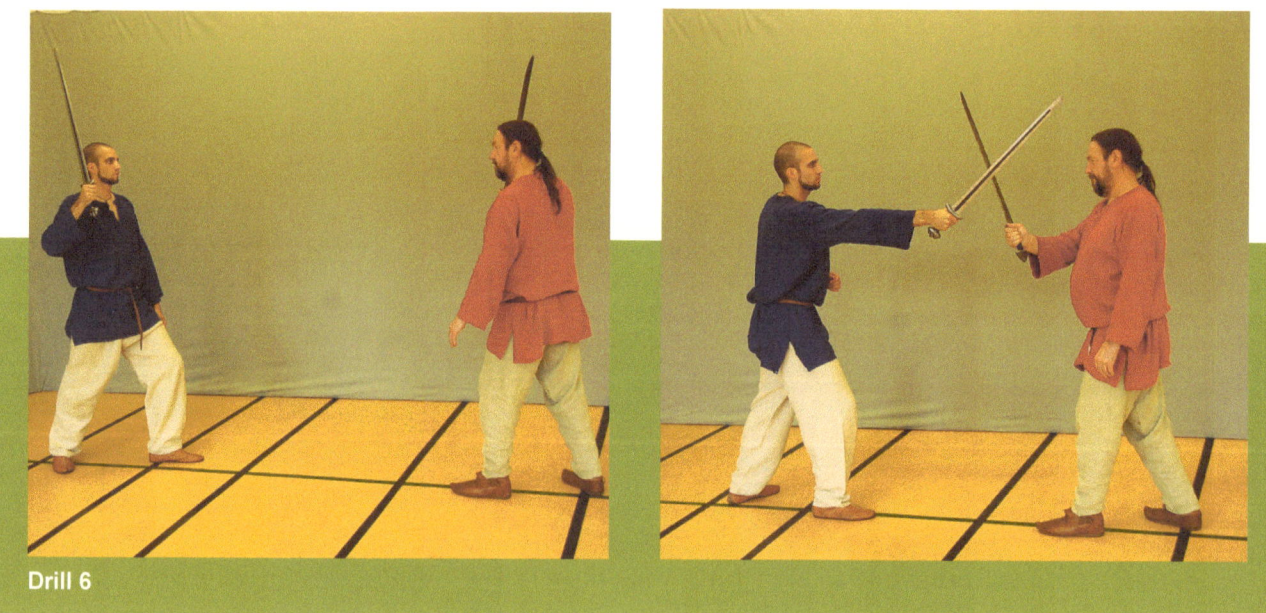

Drill 6

Blue uses attack number 1 or 2, Red parries using parry 2 to fix the opponent's sword.

Red grabs the opponent's sword pommel with the left hand.

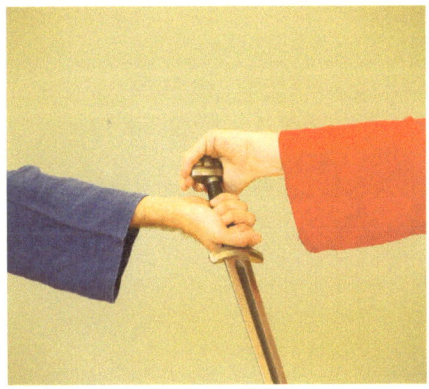

This picture shows a close up of the pommel grab, shown at a point about half way through the action.

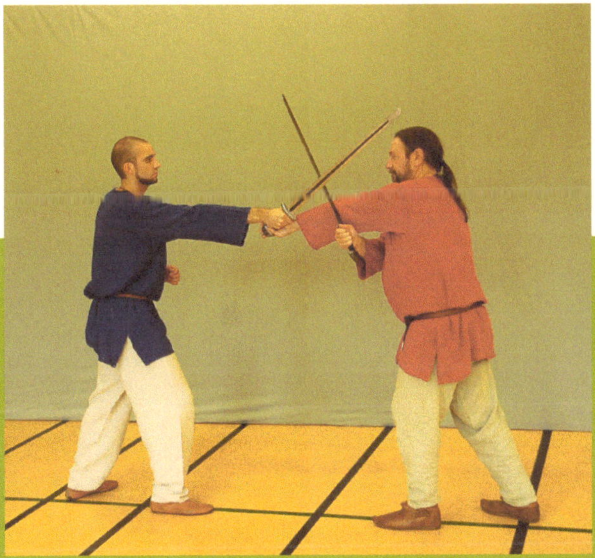

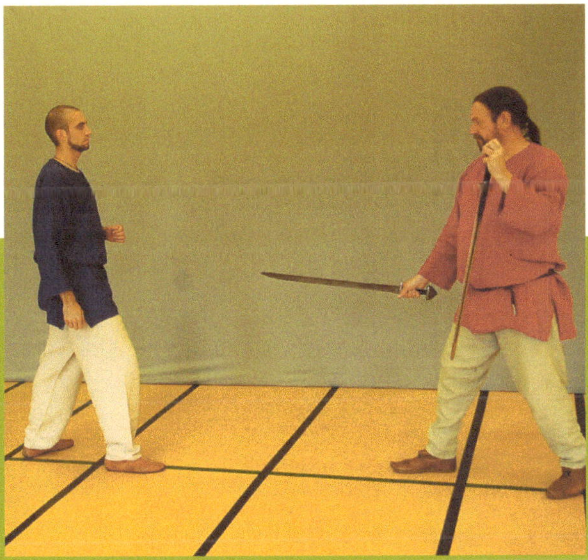

Red pulls the sword pommel towards himself, stepping backward. Extra power can be added by using the sword to push to the left.

Voilà! You have the sword.

Drill 7
Blade grab against a right handed person.

When the pommel is difficult to reach or simply not available, the alternative is to grip the blade near the handle, though anywhere will do. Simply turn the blade downward so that the handle turns either out of the front of the hand or the back as in this example. The way the blade is turned is dependent upon the initial parry made. With the use of an outside parry, the disarm can be supported by pressing down with the sword in a clockwise direction. If the parry was on the inside then the turn would be in the anti-clockwise direction and the opponent's

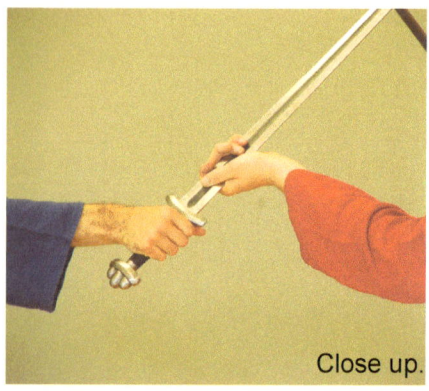
Close up.

sword would pop out of the front of the hand. In this case the left hand would lie over the right hand if the sword point was uppermost.

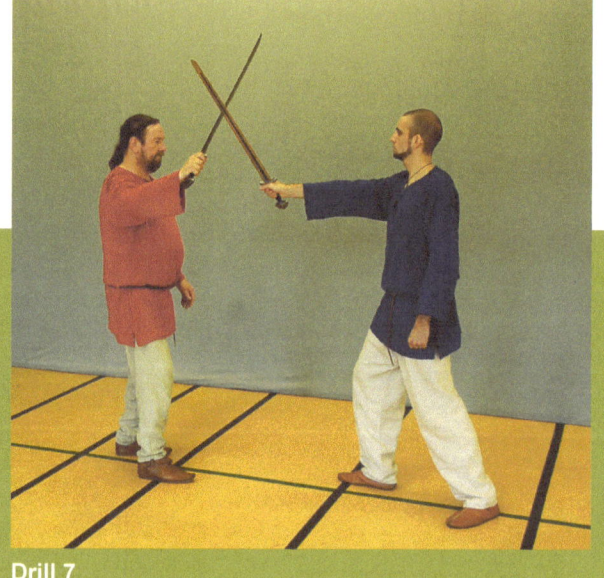
Drill 7

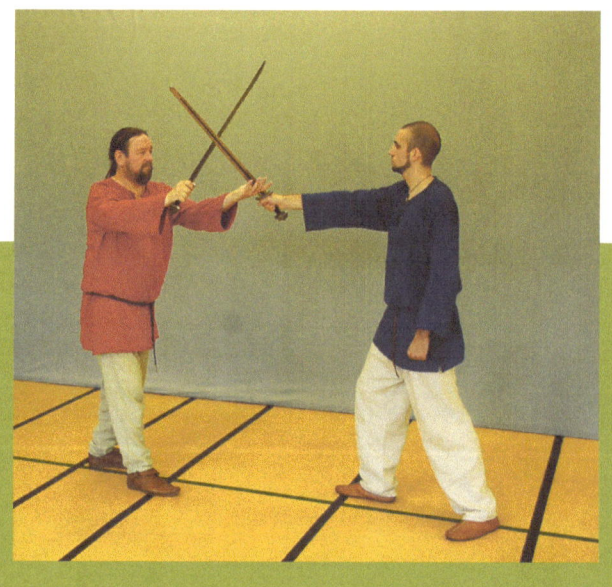

Blue uses attack number 3, Red parries using parry 2 to fix the opponent's sword.

Red with the left hand, immediately grabs the sword blade near the handle with the thumb pointing to the left. The sword can be used to help with the leverage by pushing down clockwise to the right without sliding off the opponent's blade.

This method of disarm is more often seen in stick fighting though there is absolutely no reason why they cannot be done against sharp weapons. One of the best uses in Viking era fighting is against hand axes, which can be easily disarmed using this method.

We see this blade grab time and time again in the historical treatises that deal with combat with weapons. The usual comment is that the hand will be cut after grabbing a blade. I can assure you that this does not happen with the correct technique. Not only is it possible to hold a blade without the hand touching the edge of the blade, blades normally will not cut unless they move in the hand. The technique with sharp blades is not hard to learn though we definitely do not recommend that you attempt doing this without hands on expert instruction and plenty of practice on blunt blades.

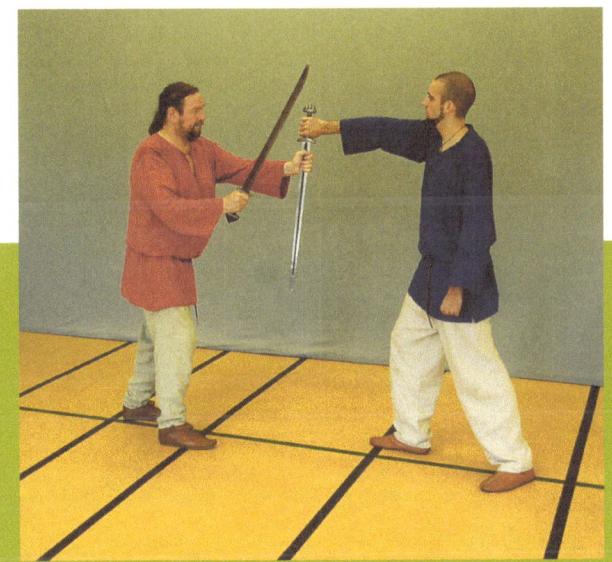
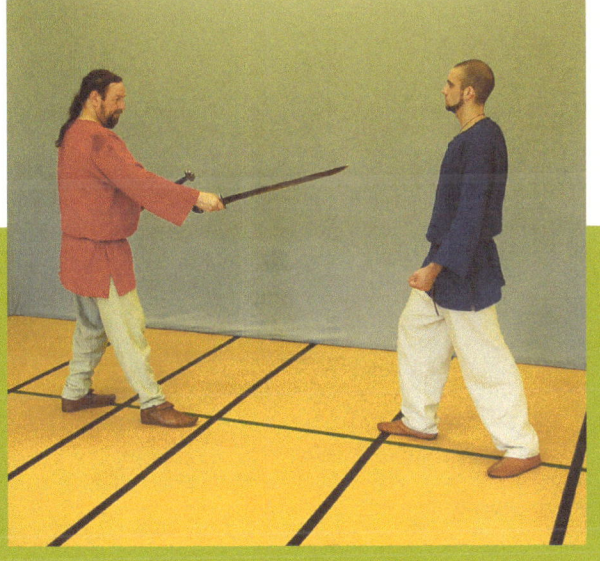

Red pulls downward turning the sword point to the floor, the turn to the left is maintained until the sword is released out of the back of the opponent's hand.

Red steps backwards with the sword in his hand.

Drill 8
Pommel grab against a right handed person by a left handed person.

Here we see the pommel grab disarm from the left handed person's perspective. After the attacker's sword has been fixed you quickly grab the pommel with the right hand and pull towards yourself, while pushing forward with the sword. As you execute the disarm you may even hit with your sword! Because of the position using opposite hands, the hand has easy access to the pommel without interfering with the sword arm, though it is easier for the opponent to intercept the arm making the disarm and stop the technique, for the same reasons.

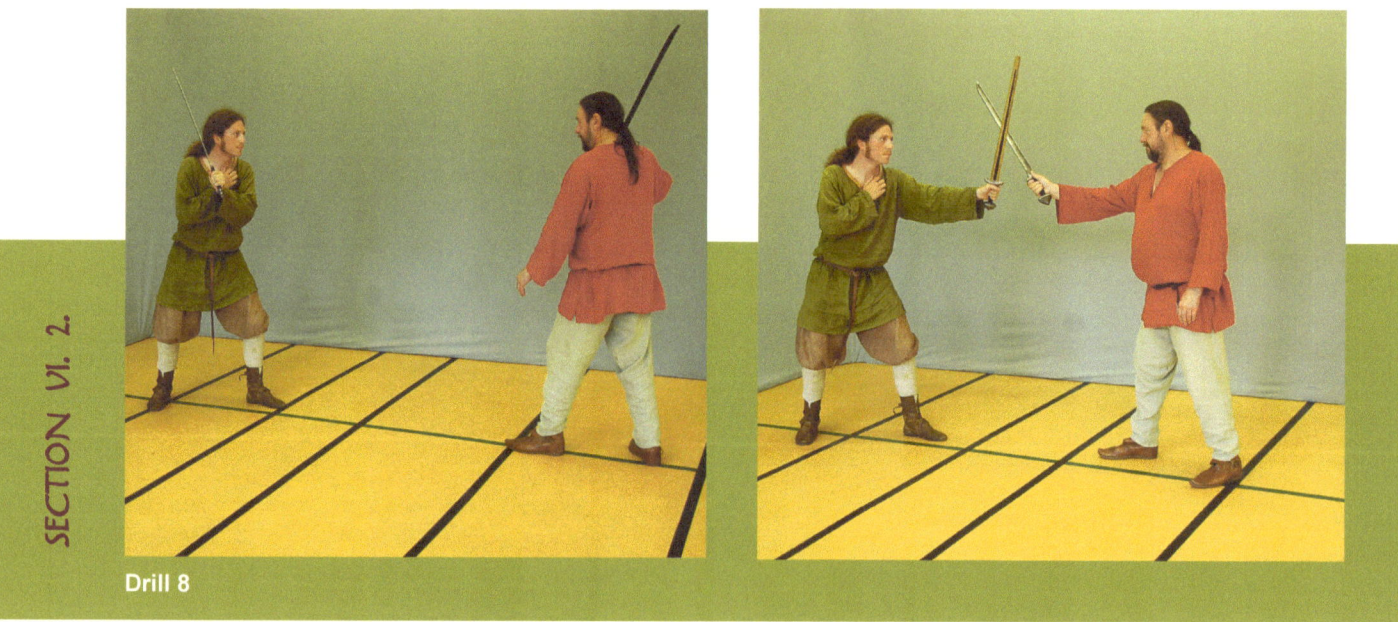

Drill 8

Red starts in guard position 2, Green in 3.

Red uses attack number 1 or 2, defender parries using parry 2 to fix the opponent's sword.

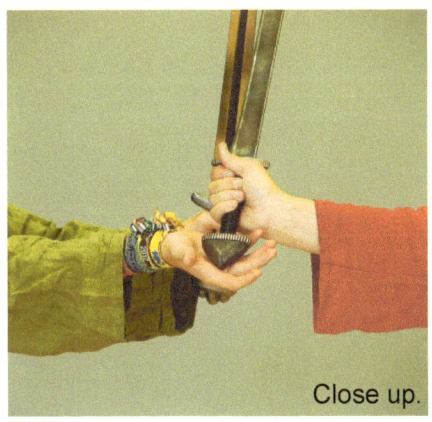

Close up.

This is extremely useful against people who linger with blade contact without actually doing something. It is worth the fighter dropping the shield if this technique can be executed.

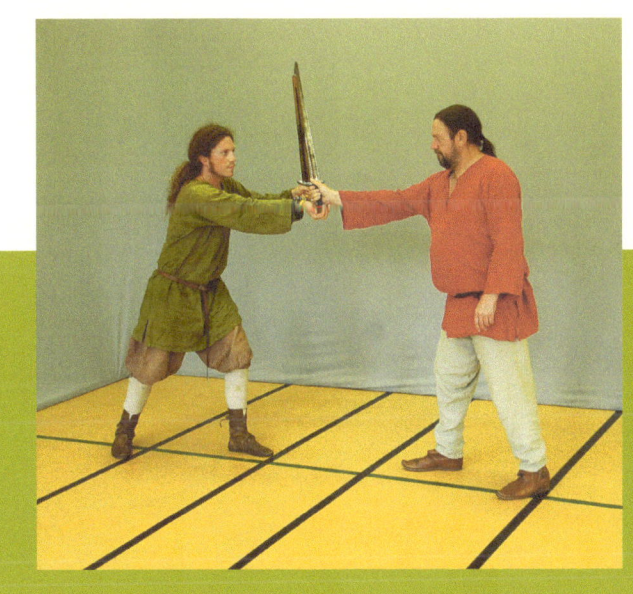

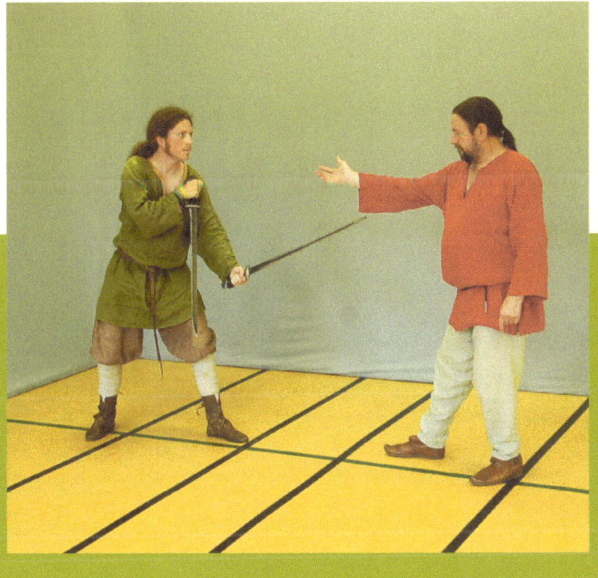

Green grips the opponent's sword pommel with the right hand.

Green pulls the sword pommel towards himself, stepping backward, while pushing forward with the sword. The sword is taken.

Drill 9
This is an example of a blade grab against a right handed person.

Likewise the left handed person can grab the blade and do the same disarm. The hand used to do the disarm goes behind the parrying hand as before, twisting downward clockwise, in this case turning also to the left until it turns out of the back of the hand. The sword aids the disarm by also pushing down and through towards the opponent, it may strike them during this movement.

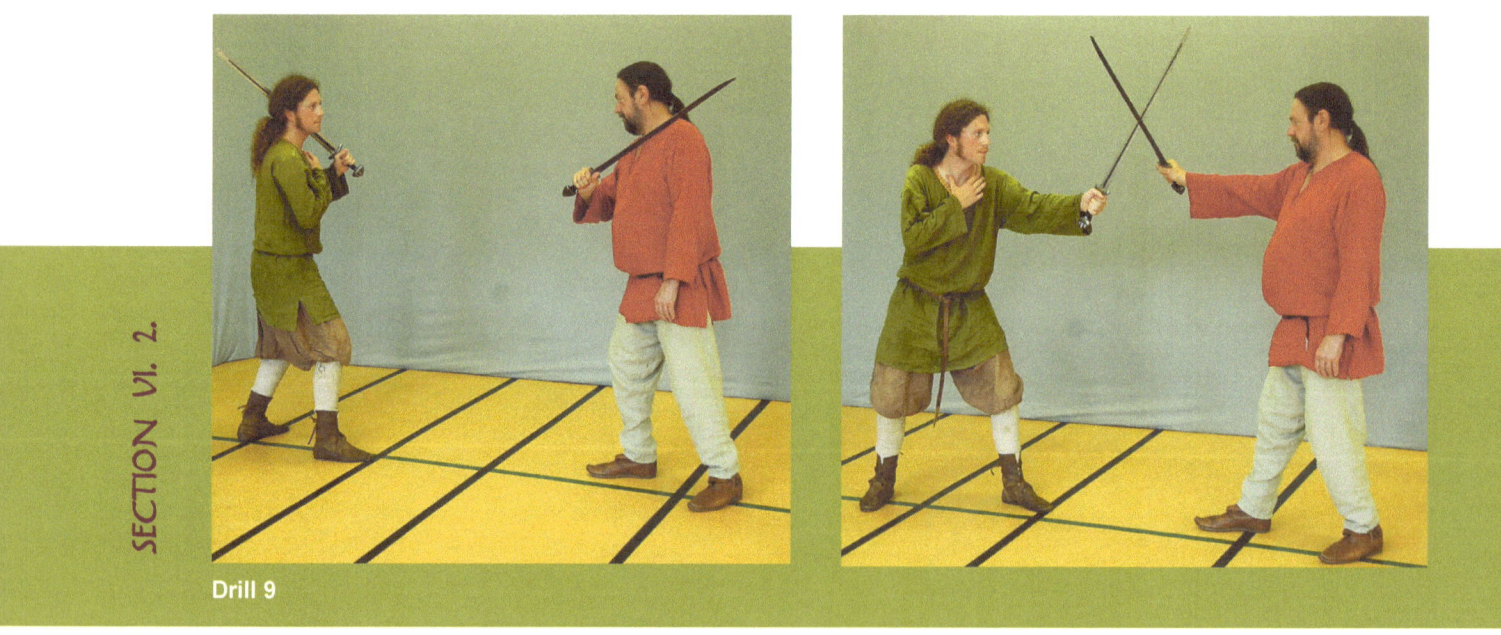

Drill 9

Red starts in position 3 and Green starts in position 2

Green uses attack number 2 and steps forward, Red parries using parry 3, making a half step back.

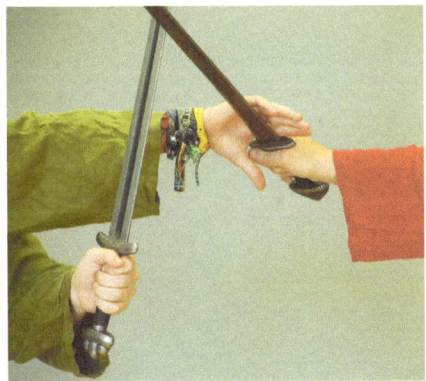

This picture shows a close up of the start of the blade grab.

This technique ends with the sword on the outside and the opponent's sword arm in the way of their own shield, not withstanding they have lost their sword. This is usually a fight winning move.

The fighter should always be aware of opportunities to disarm opponents. The more experience one has the more possibilities open up.

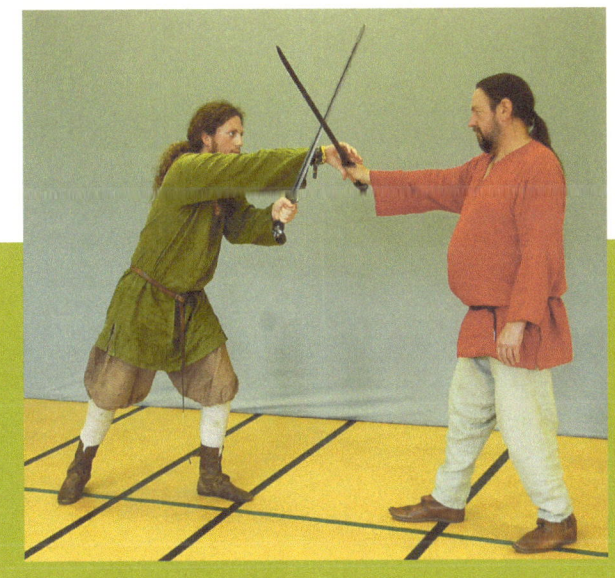

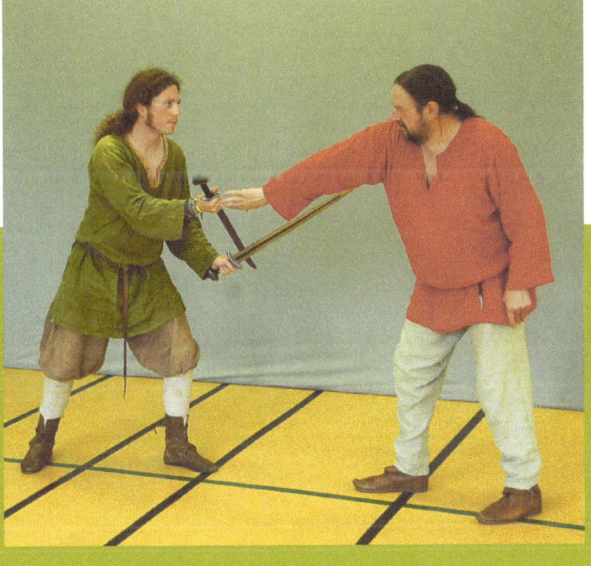

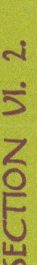

Green uses the right hand, to grab the sword blade near the grip with the thumb pointing to the left. The hand goes behind the sword blade.

Green pulls downward, turning the sword point to the floor, it is turned to the left until released out of the back of the opponent's hand. The sword is taken.

EXCHANGING THE PARRY
Drill 10-14
Exchanging the Shield for Sword

Use an invite to entice an opponent to attack the target you wish him to go for, then use the sword for the parry, you are now set up for an exchange of weapons at the parrying point. If we were going to attack with the shield, we could also exchange sword for shield, if the conditions were right. The shield is a powerful weapon of attack, as it weights maybe 3 to 6 times the weight of the sword. Striking edge on will do a great deal of damage to the opponent. It demands a great deal of control to use a shield in this way, and we will be covering this subject in more detail in the Advanced Guides. This guide will only concern ourselves with exchanging shield for the sword.

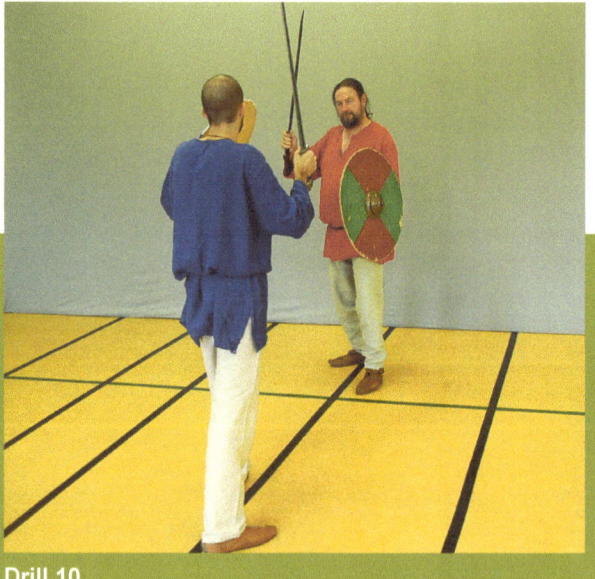

Drill 10

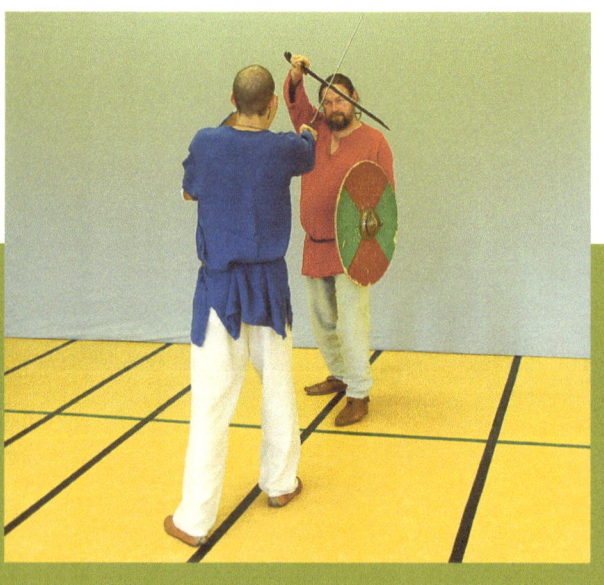

Both start in guard position 2. Blue cuts to the left shoulder.

Instead of using the shield, Red parries with the sword point down in the right Ox roof parry position. Red is now in position to exchange.

Drill 10
The initial parry is a roof block in right Ox, followed by an exchange of shield on the outside, finishing with an attack to the opponent's right shoulder.

It is important to note that the sword is not removed from the opponent's sword until the shield is in contact with the sword or the sword arm of the opponent. If the sword is moved before the shield contact then the opponent's sword is free to attack again. Remember all exchanges must be prepared by close proximity of the shield to the point of exchange almost simultaneously with the parry action.

The power of the exchange lies in the fact that when executed properly, the opponent cannot use either the sword or the shield effectively. A successful execution of this technique almost always leads to the end of the fight.

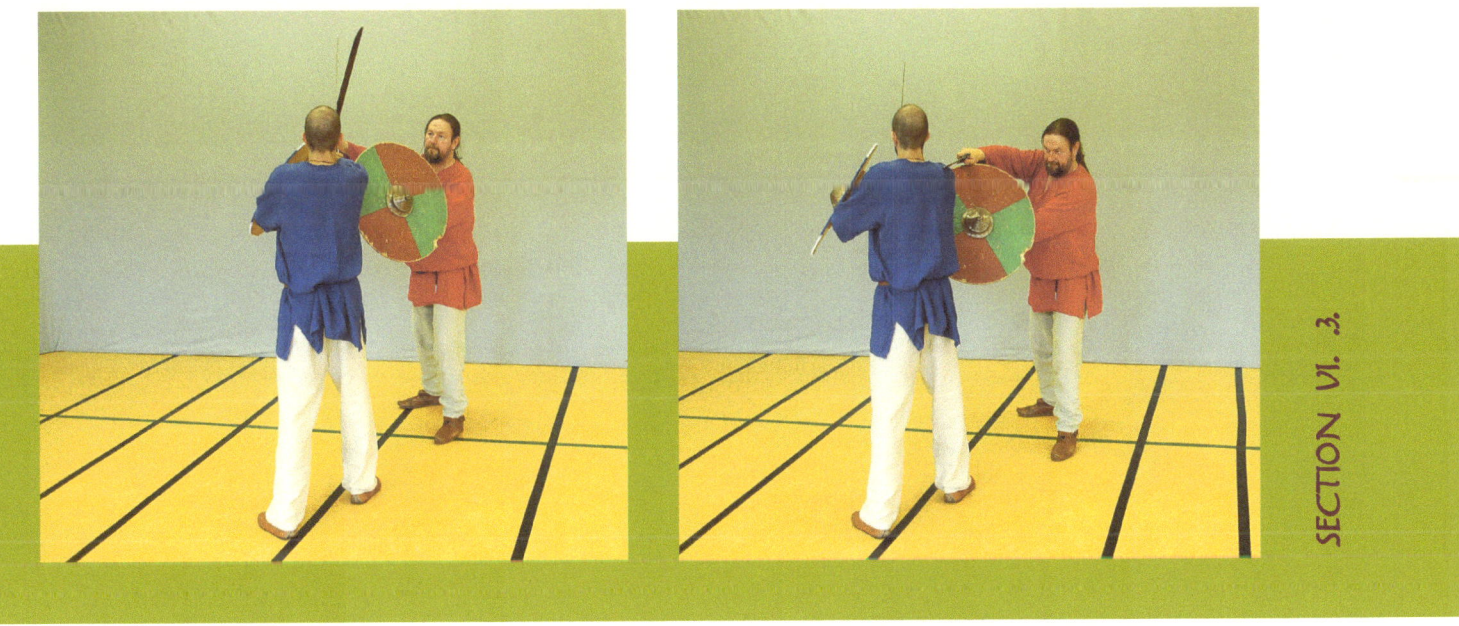

Red pushes the edge of the shield against the outside of the opponent's arm or sword to control it, the sword is released by turning the blade slightly up towards the right.

Red lands the attack on the opponent's right shoulder while stepping forward.

Drill 11
Using the sword to parry attack 2 with a roof block in right Ox, exchange shield on the inside, then attacking the opponent's right shoulder.

This exchange on the inside can open up the opponent's sword arm to a devastating cut, or you can step forward in Ox and thrust, see book 3. If Blue tries to parry the following attack with the shield using parry 3 then you could start with another combination moving to the opponent's left hand side. Such a combination would choose the left leg as the first target and could switch to others as they open up.

The inside position as shown in the picture below is an excellent place to be as leaves so many possibilities open. The counter attack can take place on the weapon arm as shown or after targeting the head it can switch to the right or left, either on the high or low line depending where the opponent places shield or sword.

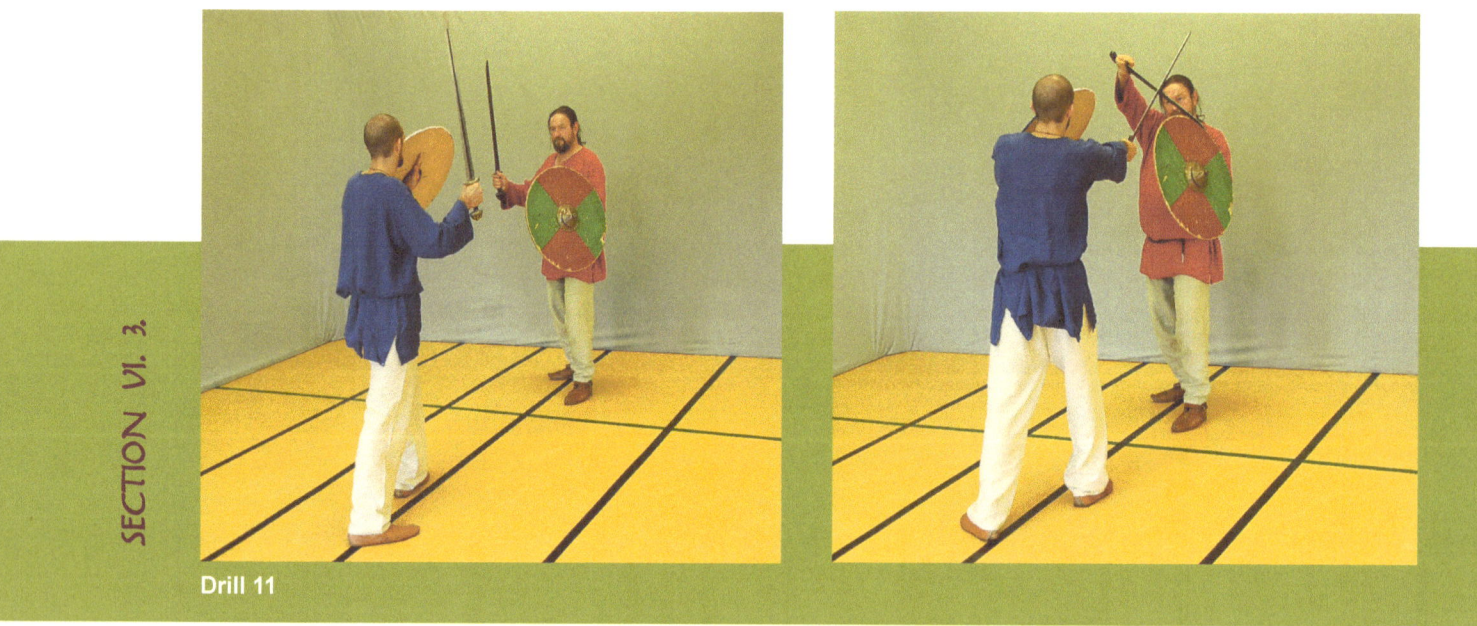

Drill 11

Both start in guard position 2. Blue attacks the left shoulder, Red needs to cover his left side.

Instead of using the shield, Red parries with the sword point down. Red is now in a position to exchange.

In the last position if blue defended the attack to the arm with the shield, Red would continue the combination by stepping diagonally to the right and cutting to the left leg of Blue from above.

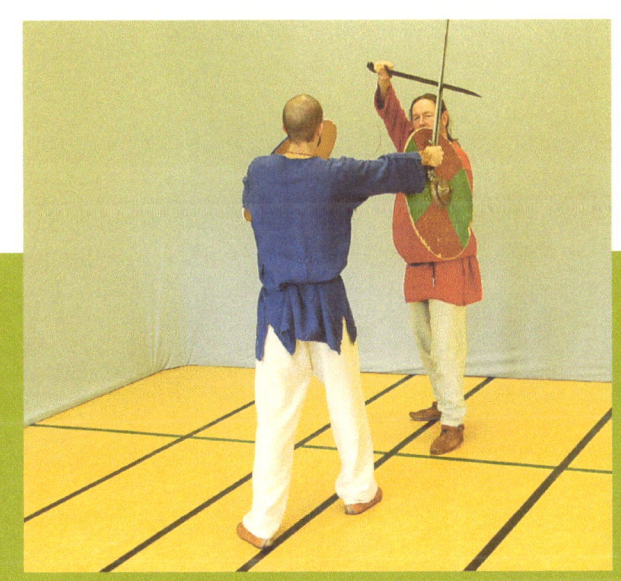 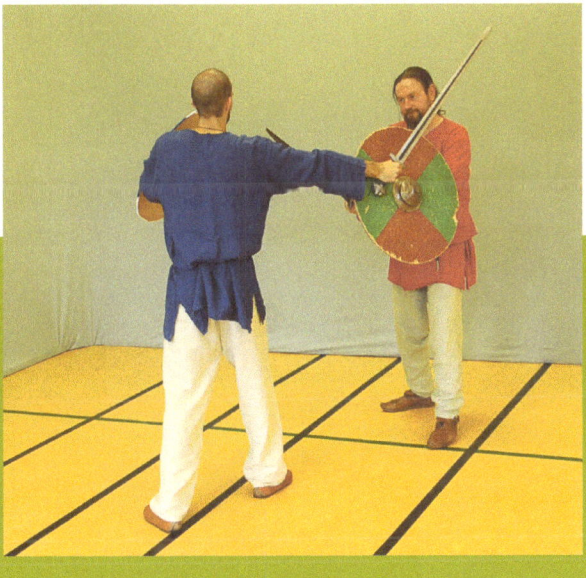

Red pushes the face of the shield against the inside of the opponent's sword or sword arm to control it and then moves it slightly to the left, releasing the sword.

Red attacks the opponent's right shoulder or arm, stepping forward as required.

Drill 12
Using the sword to execute an outside parry against attack 3, exchanging the shield on the outside, followed by attacking the opponent's right shoulder sword point down.

This is another exchange to the outside, if successful there is little that the opponent can do to stop this attack except step backward, though you can pursue easily by stepping forwards with them. You should really make this powerful sequence part of your own repertoire, by diligent practice with your partner, as there are many offshoots from this tactic.

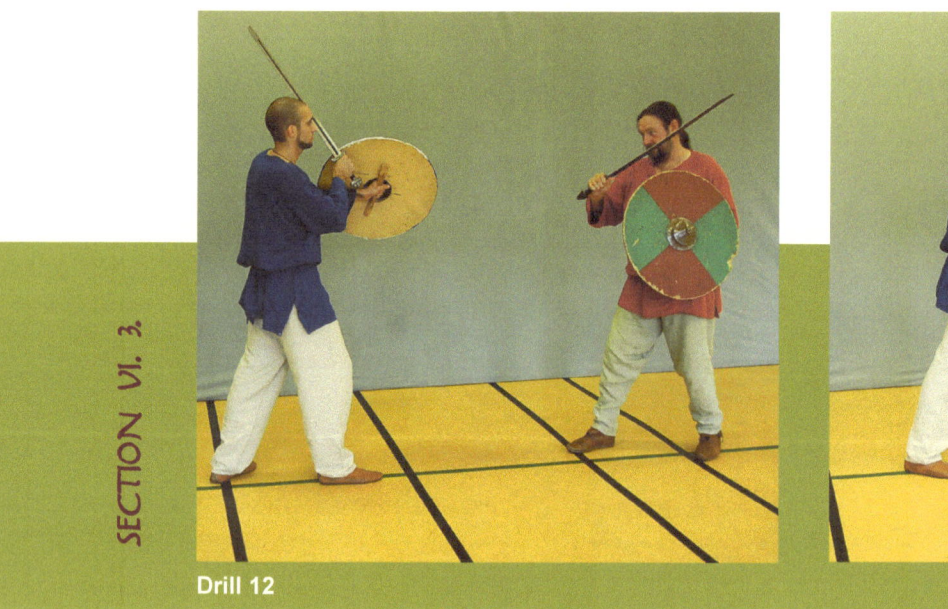

Drill 12

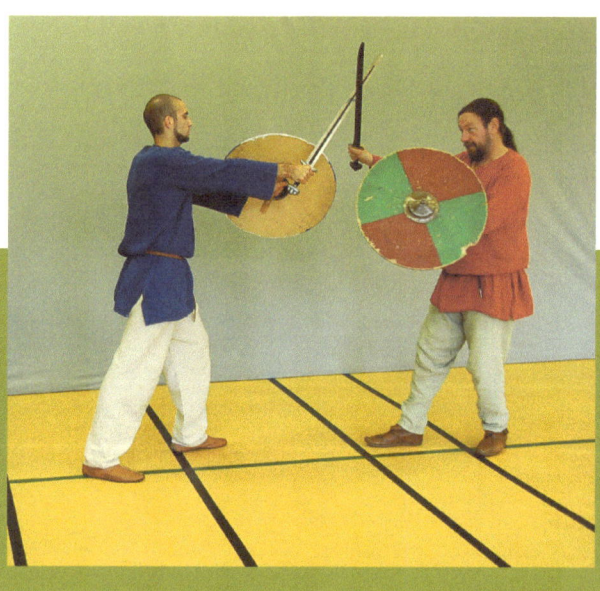

Both start in guard position 3.

Blue cuts to the right shoulder after making a full step. Red, instead of using the shield, parries with the sword point up. Red is now in a position to exchange.

Notice that Blue's sword is controlled by both Red's sword and shield until the point where Red starts the counter attack. This is key to the whole technique sequence, this feeling of having his sword controlled by the opponent, will in many cases undermine Blue's resolve, and put increasing pressure on him, leading to mistakes.

Should Blue step backwards, Red should pursue though step diagonally to the right, in this case Blue's head should be open; if this line is defended by the shield, then Red should follow the line of the shield down to the left leg which at this point will be forward below the shield. This continuation of another combination makes the opponent's job even more difficult.

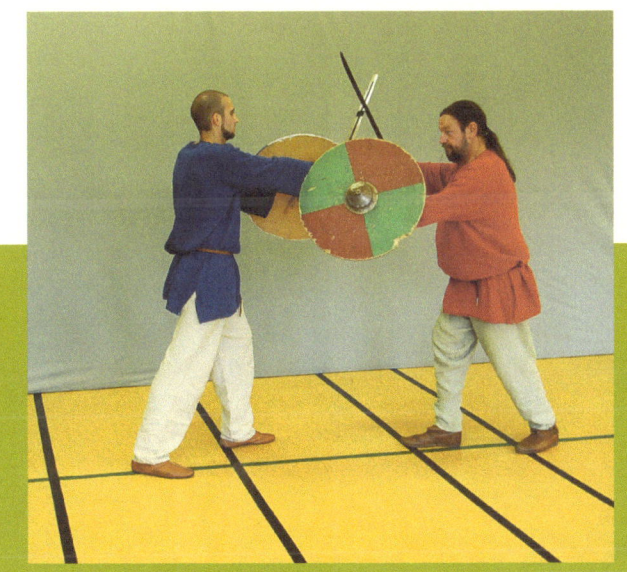

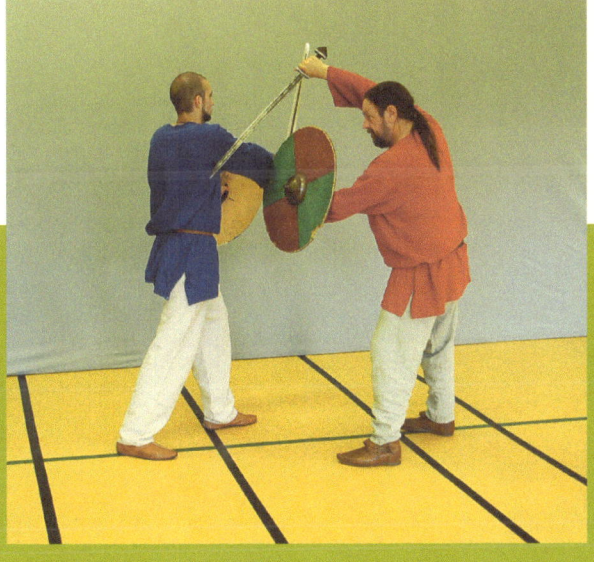

Red pushes the edge of the shield against the outside of the opponent's arm or sword to control it, releasing the sword.

Red makes a diagonal step to the left with the left leg and cut down onto the opponent's sword arm with the point down.

Drill 13
Beginning with a sword parry on the inside against attack 4, make a shield exchange on the inside, finishing with an attack to the opponent's left thigh.

It is possible to exchange even if the attack is low, though it is not so easy and requires practice. The shield face may have to turn be turned down a little so that the opponent's sword cannot just slip over the face and into the shoulder. This should not happen if the parry caught the sword underneath the boss as occurs in the third picture. The transfer to the opponent's left hand side is easy though note that the control of the opponent's sword will be lost as this move is made. This is not so much of a disadvantage as this is also a move away from the opponent's weapon. With an exchange on the inside the fighter should dominate the centre or be able to slip to the opponent's left hand side easily.

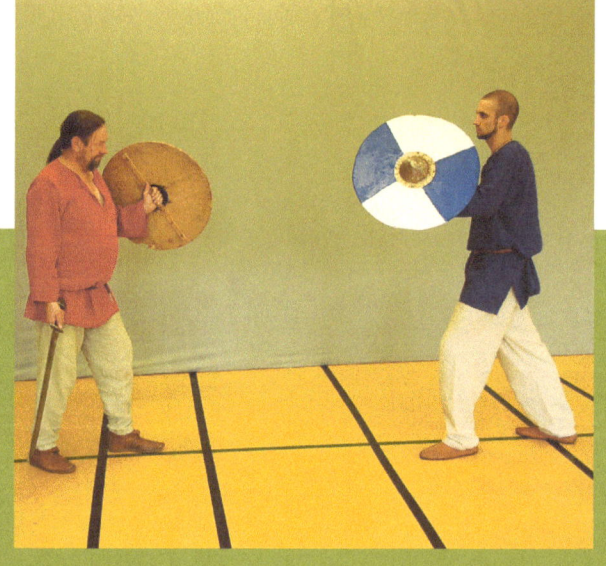

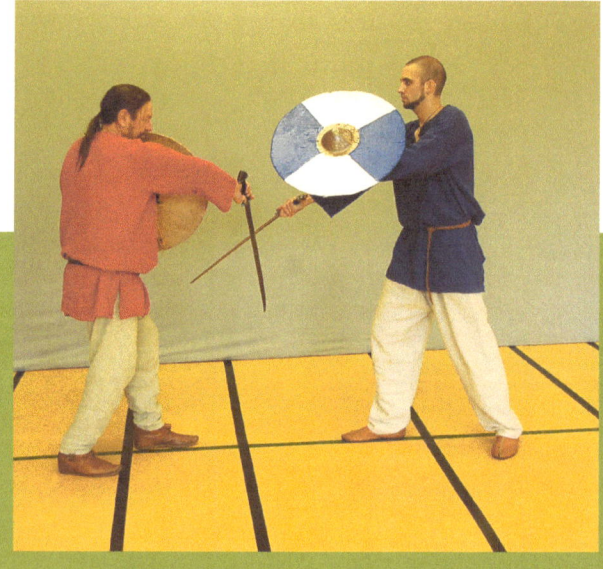

Both start in guard position 4.

Blue cuts to the left thigh from below, after making a full step, Red must parry low on the left using sword parry 4.

As the exchange takes place it may be possible for Red to attack the sword arm of the opponent. This would usually intimidate Blue to use the shield to prevent this, then if Red switches to the right side Blue's left leg may be even more open.

If Blue swings the left leg behind the right to turn to face the forward leg can become the target. If Blue does not materially alter the distance, he will be just as open under the shield.

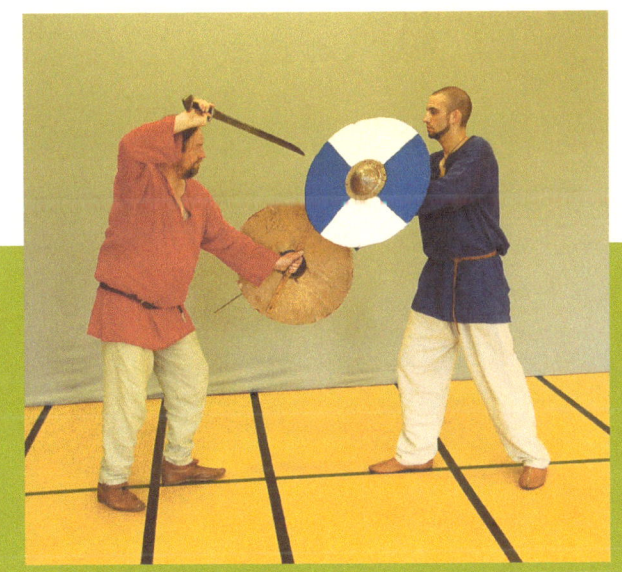

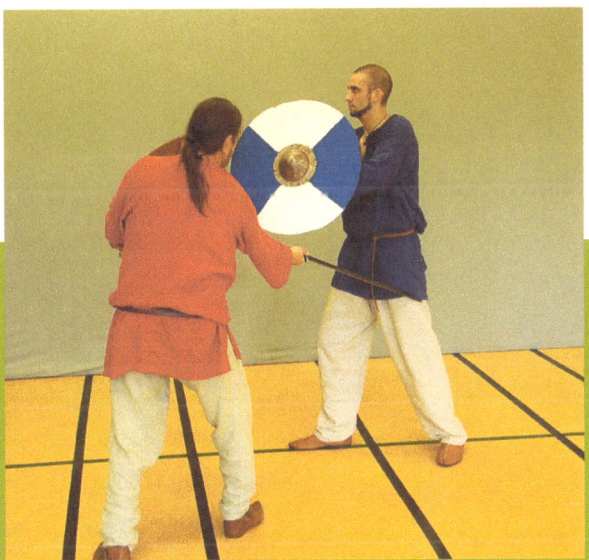

Red pushes the edge of the shield against the inside of the opponent's sword arm to control it and then pushes it to the left, releasing the sword.

Red attacks the opponent's left thigh from below, though this could also be from above, while stepping diagonally forward to the right.

Drill 14
Starting with sword parry 5 against attack 5, exchange shield on the outside, followed by attacking the opponent's right shoulder.

Here Red parries with the sword is on the outside, and as with all outside parries they are much easier to exchange weapons on the outside because that is the actual current situation. It is possible to exchange weapons that have initially contacted on the inside on the outside, though this requires special circumstances. One instance where this can happen is when the opponent's strike is strong at the point of contact, if you can feel this strength at contact you can redirect the force out towards your outside, thereby allowing an exchange of weapons. This topic is covered briefly in book 3. This drill is a classic swap of a sword parry on the outside, with a shield on the outside. It is a powerful sequence and should be studied well.

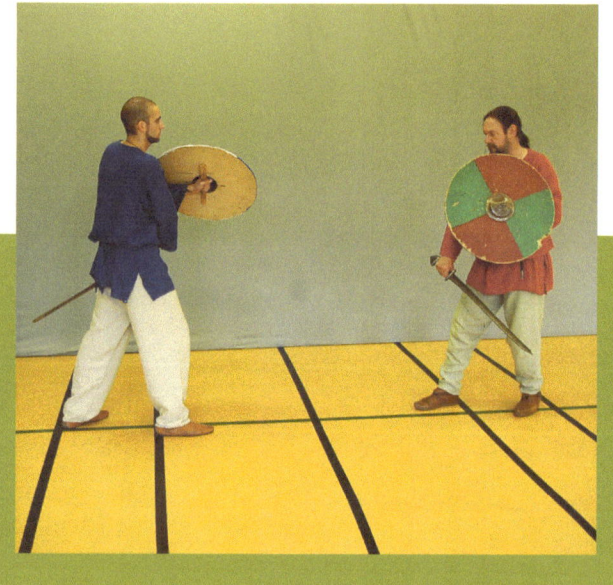

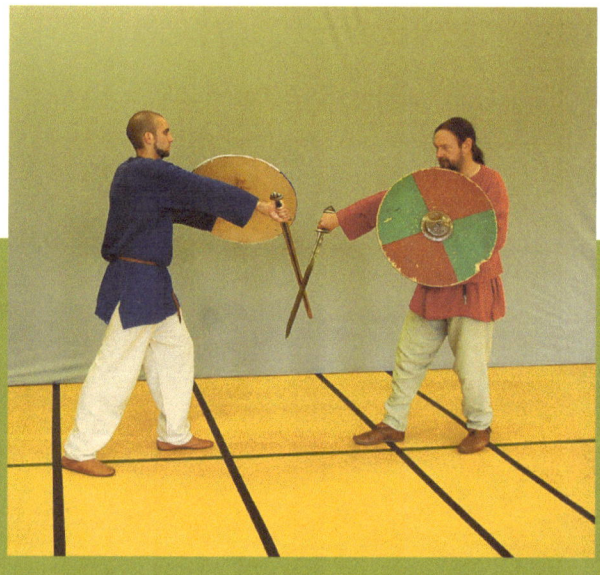

Both fighters are in guard position 5. Blue cuts for Red's right thigh.

Red parries with sword parry 5 instead of the shield, while stepping back with a half step. Red is now in position to exchange.

Notice again that Blue's sword is contacted by both of Red's weapons at the point of exchange. This means that at no point in the exchange process is the opponent's weapon free from contact. For Blue to free his sword from this position will, even if successful, usually lead to an awkward situation where further defence is difficult.

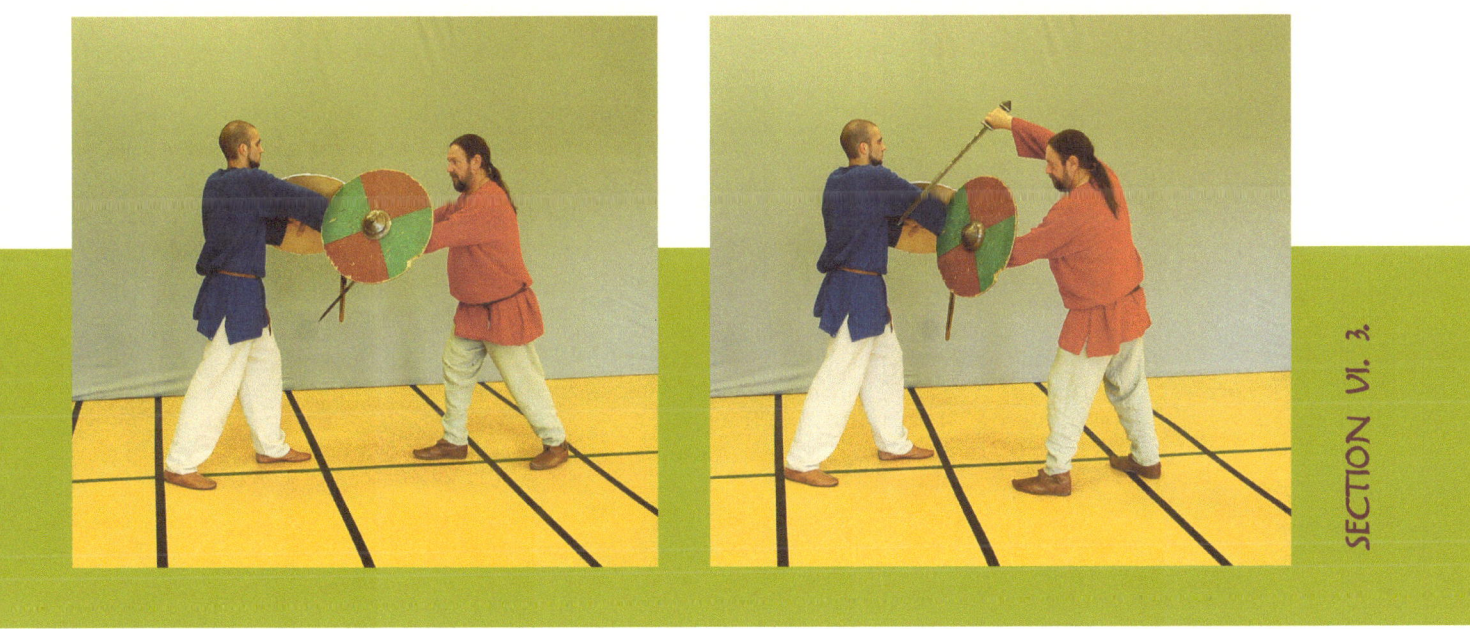

Red exchanges shields on the outside, by pressing the shield against the arm or sword, releasing the sword.

Red steps a full step diagonally forward to the left and attacks Blue's arm with the sword point down.

SECTION VII – CONCLUSION

COMMON ERRORS

As usual we conclude the book with a brief look at common errors that we have seen people make time and time again and also an example of a fight sequence.

Errors are unavoidable in combat, that is a fact. Training and practice are designed to reduce the number of errors that occur by programing the correct response into the muscle memory of the person. The errors that we showcase in these pictures are really gross errors that people should try to eradicate right from the start of the learning process. Combat should be elegant and these errors just spoil the whole picture as soon as they occur.

Note that it is the principle behind the picture that is important. The principle can be applied to all similar circumstances not just those depicted. For example in picture 1 we see a cramped position, with arms collapsed against the body. Cramped positions are almost always bad in weapon combat. See picture 5 below.

In the second picture, fully stretched positions are over extended and therefore unstable and open to numerous counters.

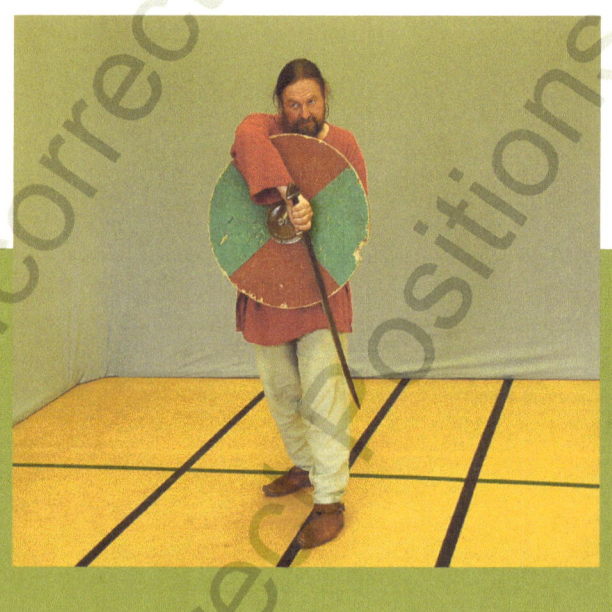

Common Error 1
Striking with the sword in front of the shield at close distance. This allows the opponent to press in with his shield and pin your sword to your shield effectively making your weapons useless.

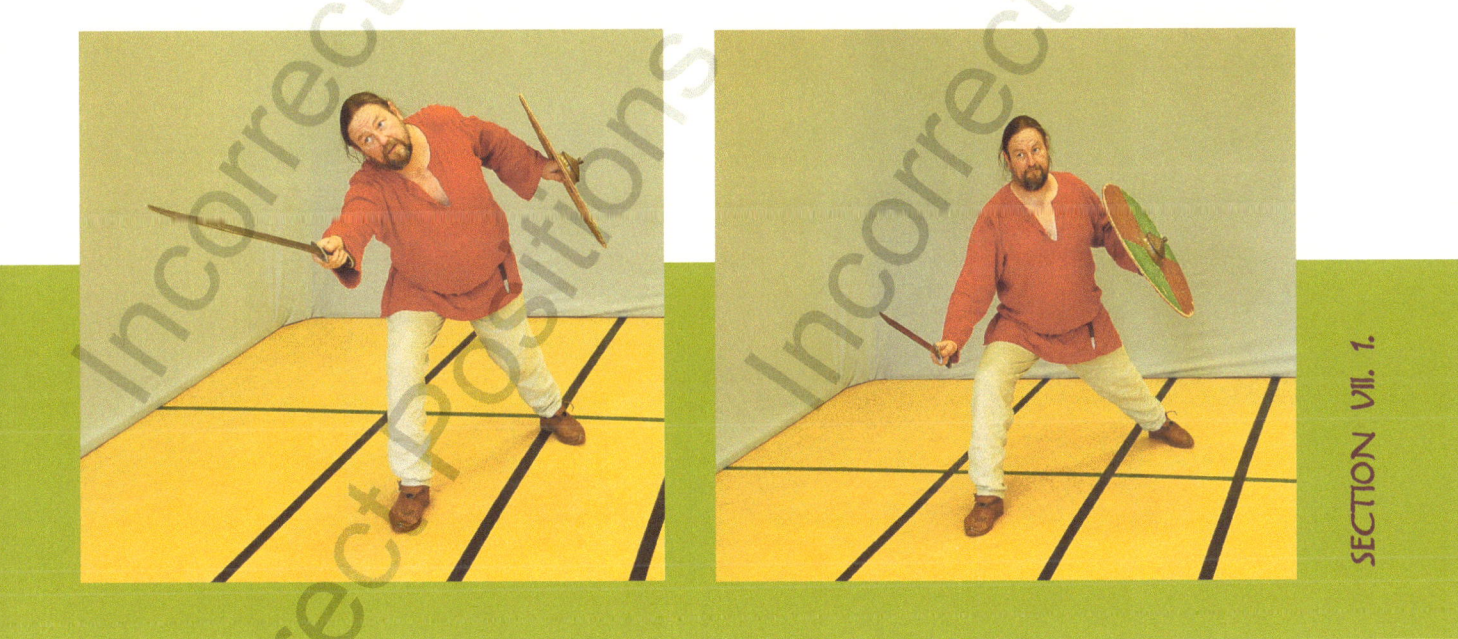

Common Error 2
Reaching too far to hit the target, is very poor technique. This position is vulnerable in so many ways, parrying is not easy, you can be pulled over forwards, and pushed over from the side and recovery to the normal stance is slow. Notice the unused shield and the forward position of the body.

Common Error 3
Stepping outside the shoulder width if on wet or slippy terrain. This is similar to the previous mistake, plus you are extremely likely to slip and fall in a way that is not easy to recover from.

Common Error 4

Dropping the sword back to swing is a waste of time and energy. Not only does it waste time, it is also a great signal of intent to the opponent. Sword attacks and parries should go from the start position to the target without any other movement.

Common Error 5

Exchanging a sword with a shield at the wrong distance. This position is too cramped and too near. Exchanging takes some time to do, it is possible for the opponent to disengage quickly and then find all your targets very near and easy to hit. The structure has also been lost from the guard position and therefore the strength.

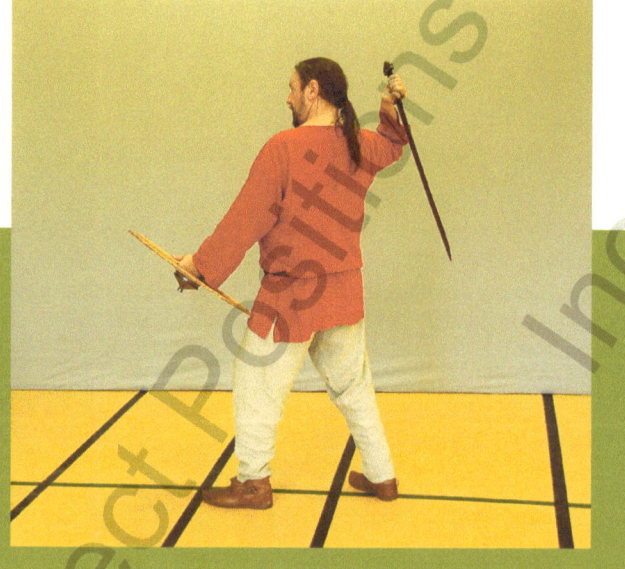
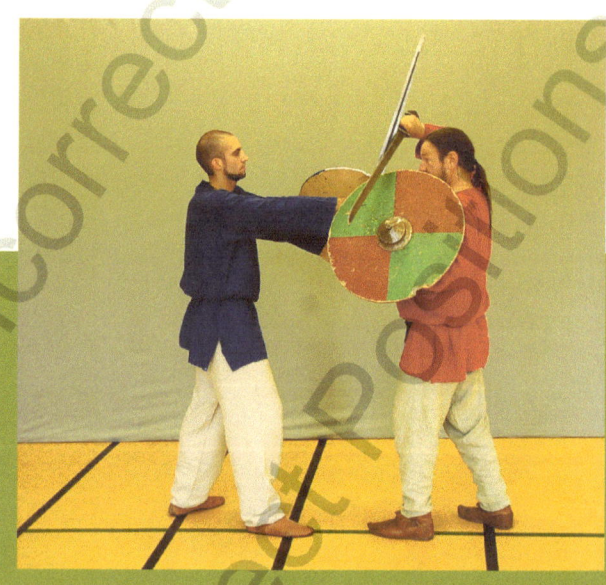

Common Error 6
Stepping too far to the side while making a counter attack. This is simply an experience problem, after you have trained sufficiently this sort of misjudgment of distance becomes less and less.

Common Error 7
Making a Roof Parry with the point to the side or angled backwards. This can lead to the sword hand or arm being hit because they are very exposed in this position. This can only be done if your parry is very late, so that the opponent cannot redirect the blade to the hand. Sometimes opponent's only strike to shields and swords because they are afraid of hurting the other combatant, these opponent's are not good to train with repeatedly because they will pose no threat and partner will also learn bad habits.

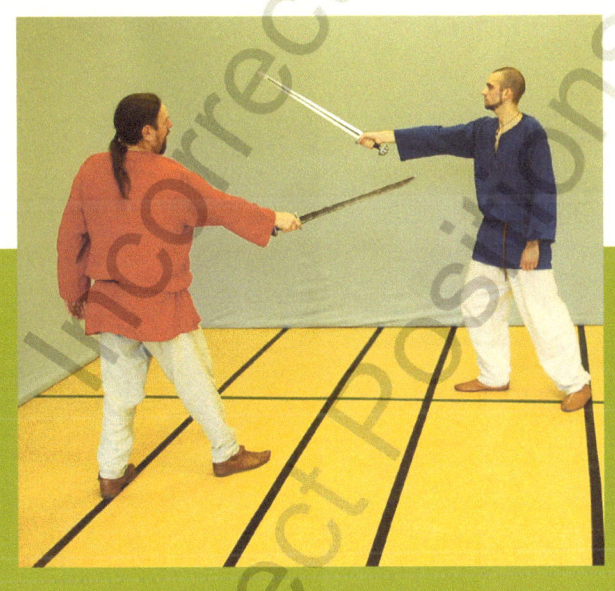
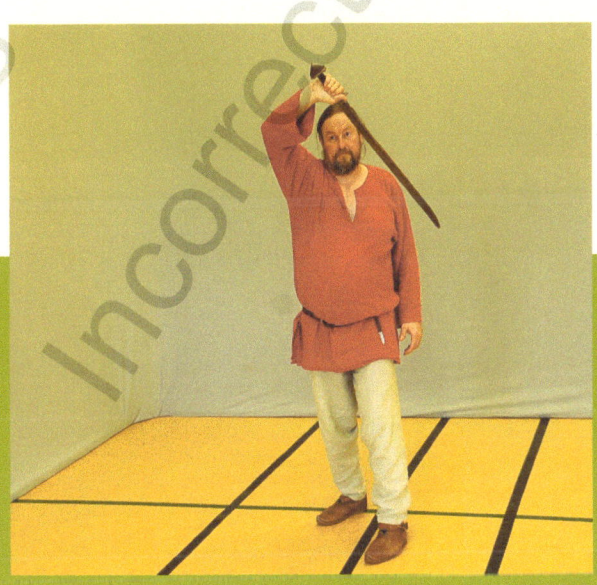

AN EXCHANGE OF BLOWS
A SAMPLE COMBAT

We now present a short sequence as an example of how a fight can progress. All fights in which the opponents are evenly matched tend to develop along the lines of attack and counter attack, as the initiative flows from one fighter to the next. How this progression takes place depends upon the fighting styles of the combatants, the tricks they like to try and the overall situation. Some people prefer fighting on flat ground, others like woods and grass, or even just in the training hall.

Speed of movement plays a part though far more important is timing and control. When the timing of a movement is correct the speed that people are moving at is mostly irrelevant. Gaining control of the opponent's weapons or positioning your body correctly at the correct time forces the opponent to attempt counters that are technically inferior.

It is important also to persevere and be willing to repeat a technique, maybe in a slightly different form or on the other side so that you gain the experience of making technique during the rigors of the fight.

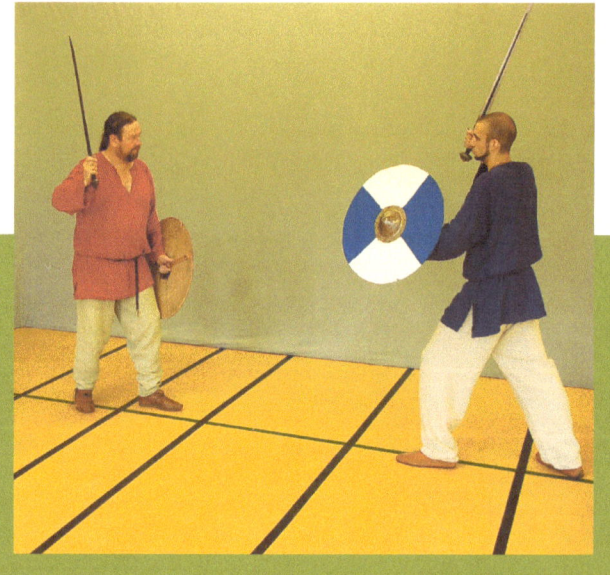

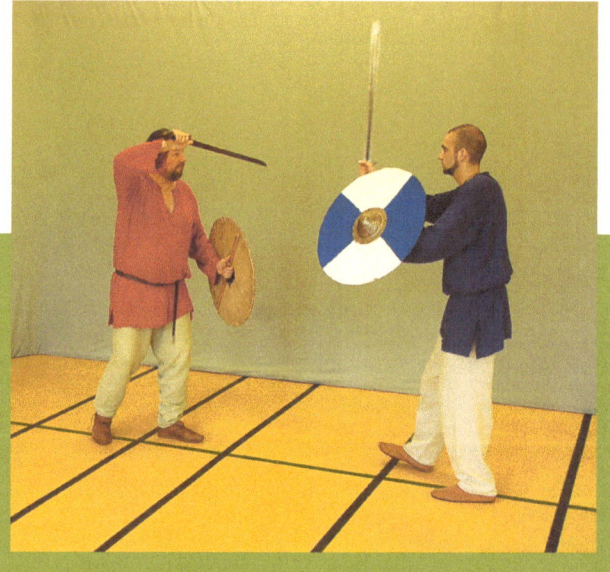

Red stands in right ox, Blue stands in guard position 2.

Blue steps forward and attacks Red's left shoulder which is open. Red prepares a roof block while simultaneously stepping forwards off line.

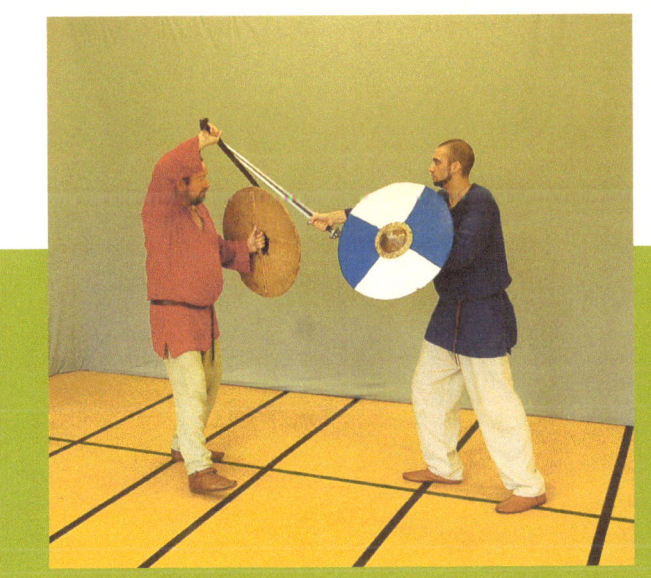 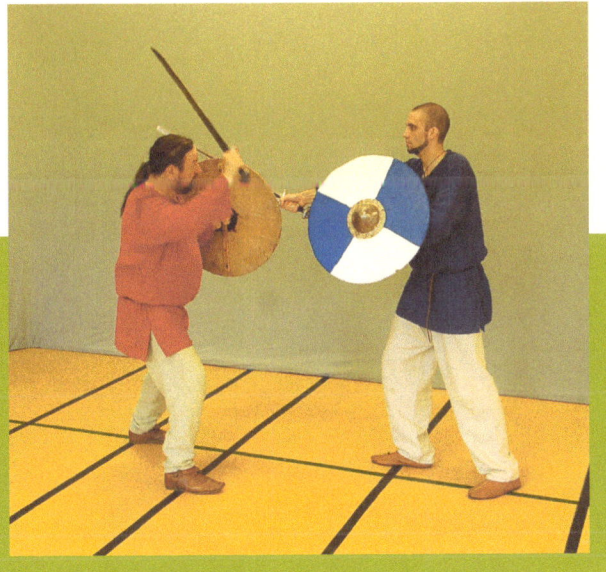

Red steps diagonally forward to the right, and makes a right Ox roof block parry. Note that Red's shield is directly behind the sword for added safety and to prepare the exchange of sword for shield.

Red releases his sword by exchanging it with his shield. Red continues moving and makes a small diagonal half step further to the right.

Red makes a cut from below against the left thigh of Blue, which Blue intercepts with the face of the shield.

Blue decides to also go under the shield of Red but to try and bring Red's shield higher he lifts his sword blade as a kind of feint.

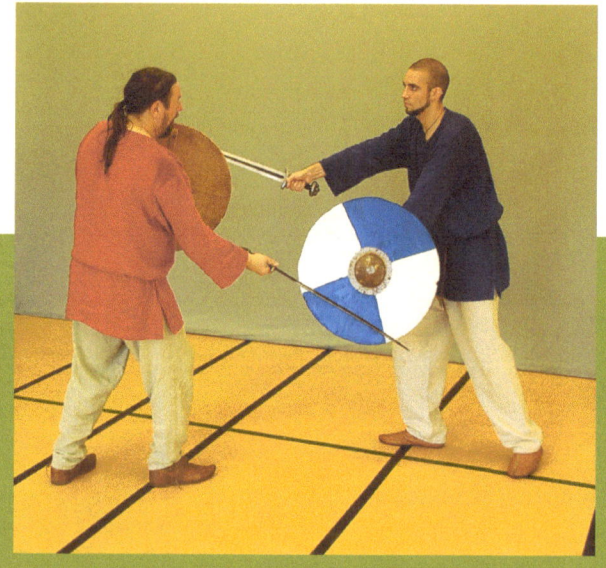
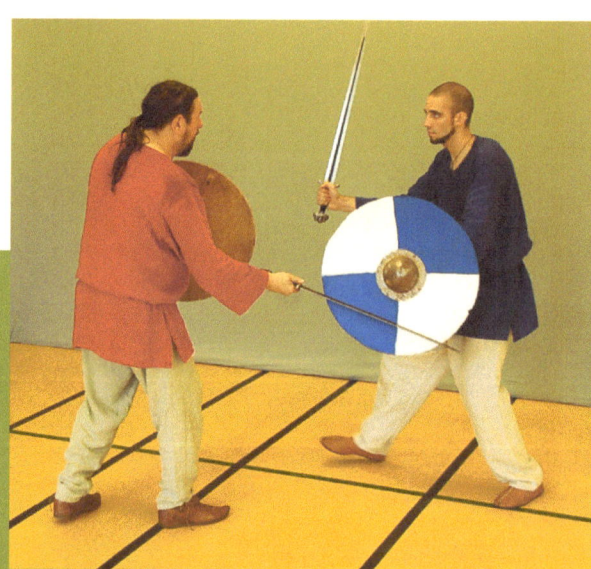

SECTION VII. 2.

Red is not fooled by this sword manoeuvre as his shield is fairly centrally placed and he does not need to move it until late. Red sees that Blue's sword arm is now exposed, lifts his sword also. Blue responds by raising his own shield quite high, Red instantly decides that the best chance is to re-attack Blue's legs.

Blue sees the danger in time and lowers his shield face to make the parry. Red starts to step backwards to move away from Blue's sword.

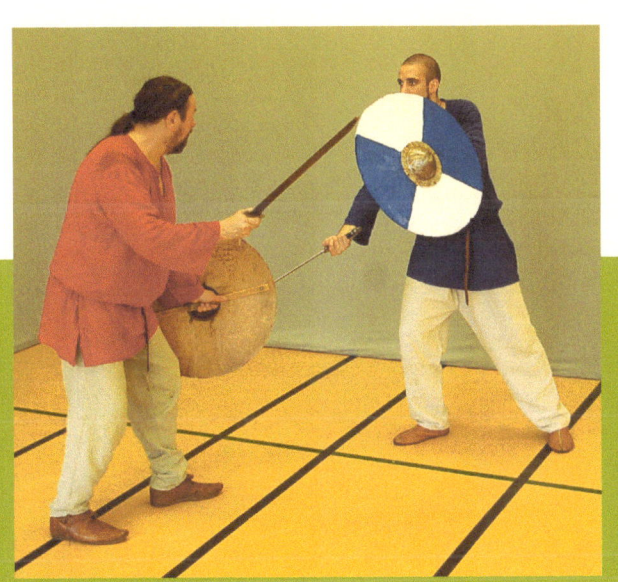
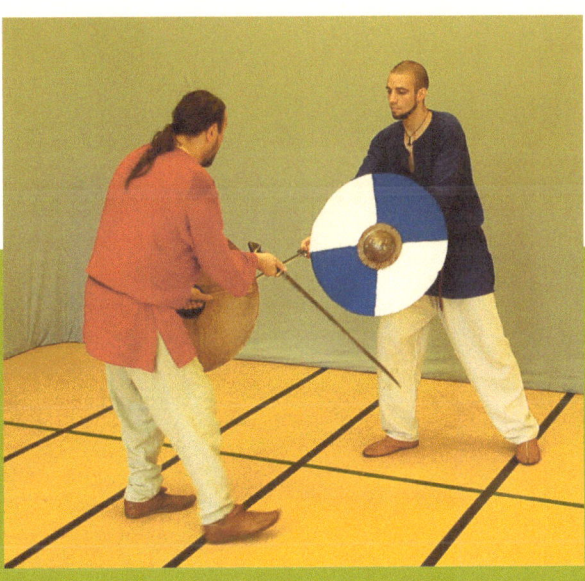

Red has finished his manoeuvre and Blue has parried the threat with his shield.

Red does not wish to lose the initiative now so he tries a difficult move and makes a diagonal transition from the lower left to the upper right of the opponent. Blue's upper sword arm is exposed.

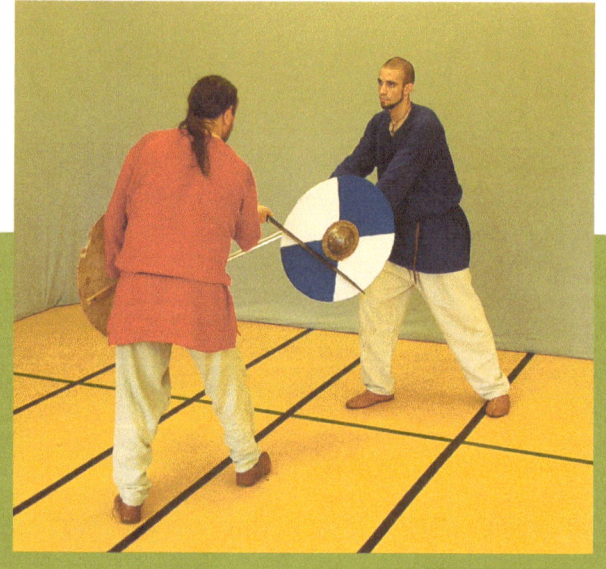 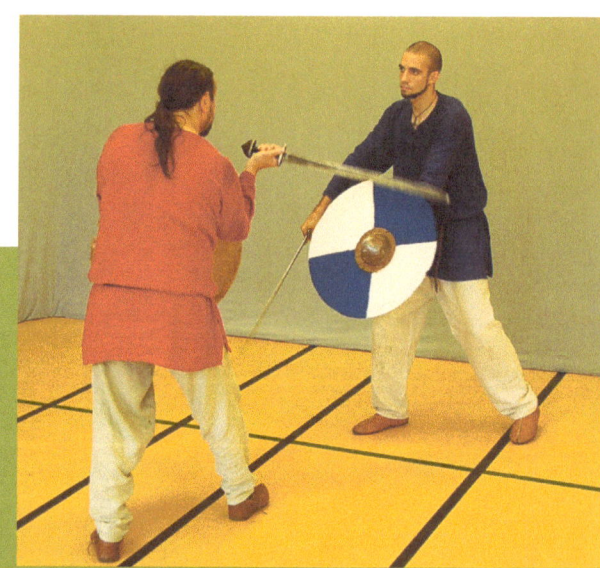

SECTION VII. 2.

Red has to move across the whole front of Blue to execute the cut. Usually this is best done if the opponent's concentration is lowered, or they are tired or out of position, Blue is neither of these in this position. Red is trying to overwhelm his opponent, unfortunately he does not show proper caution as is caught exposed in the middle of this manoeuvre.

Blue parried the attack with his sword with the right Ox Roof Parry and while stepping diagonally back away from the attack simultaneously raising his shield to exchange on the outside. This is a really bad situation for Red.

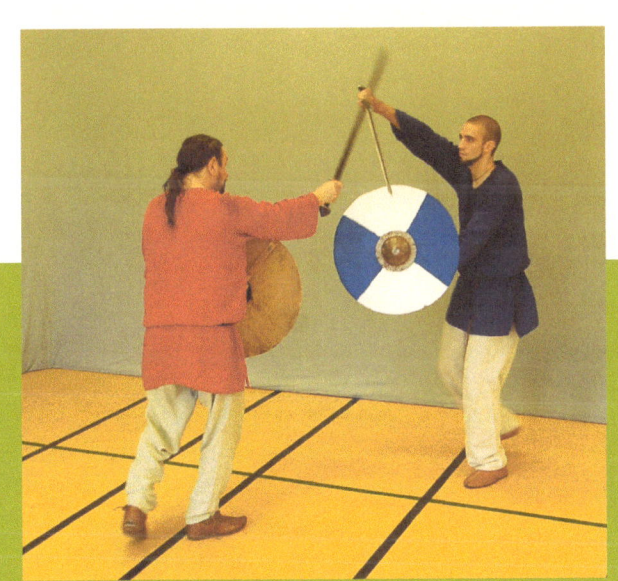
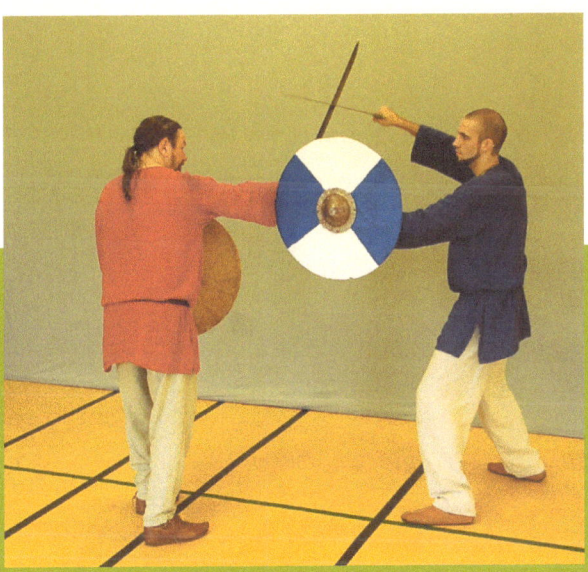

This is a classic situation, one fighter gains the initiative and maintains it for some time, their confidence grows until they push too far and try to exploit an opening that does not really exist. Red's final sequence was only a fanciful attempt to land the blow, the opponent's sword arm was not really a target, and should have been left alone. Red could have let the initiative slip to the opponent or continued to pressure Blue on his shielded side by moving to the right until Blue made a mistake. The lesson to be learned from this is that no matter who has the initiative, the correct tactical sequence must be maintained and the technique correctly executed or disaster can happen in what might have looked like a promising situation. Pushing too hard to achieve the win is just as bad as missing easy opportunities, and this is how many fights play out. Defence is harder to learn though good defence is absolutely essential if you wish to be effective: Never neglect defence at the expense of attack!

SECTION VII. 2.

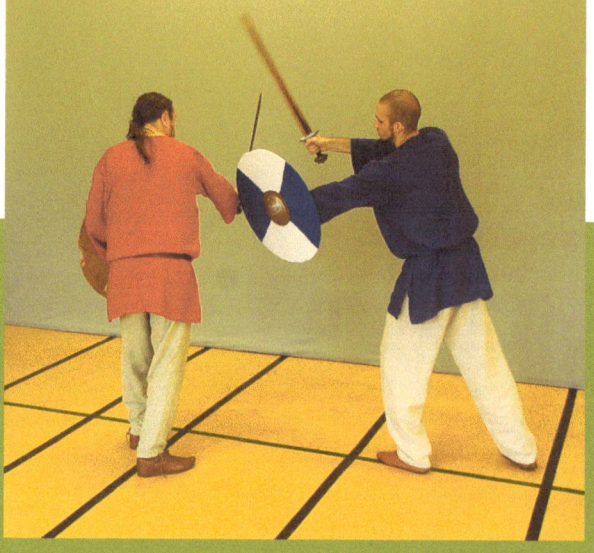

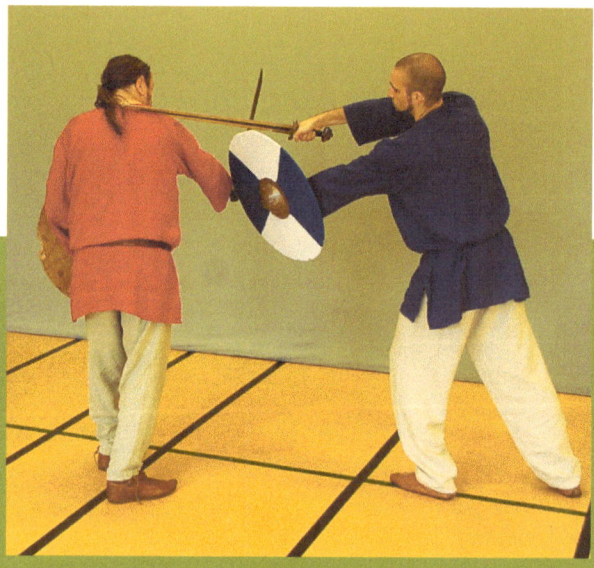

Blue exchanges the shield for the sword, pushing in with the shield and turning Red.

Blue finishes the technique with a cut from above to Red's shoulder. This ends the fight.

CONCLUSIONS

The main challenge for the student learning from these books is to develop the drills and exercises in a way which best complements their own fighting style. Each drill can be modified in many ways and also combined with others to produce a completely different set of drills. The only problem is not to make them too complicated so that the theme is lost.

We suggest that three to four movements are enough to learn unless the drill is a flow drill which just repeats the same movements in a cycle, something we will cover in later material. These movements can contain any element that the student has so far learned and can swing from attack to counter attack as required.

There is much more to learn and the best way to learn is to find a competent instructor to guide your training. Look out for seminars in your area presented by Colin Richards and also our online learning program hopefully starting in 2014. Keep in touch on our web site and Facebook page and send us your comments and suggestions.

Please remember, whatever use you put this information to, that control and safety are of prime concern. We wish you a pleasant and rewarding experience in the world of historical European Viking combat.

SECTION VII. 3.

FURTHER MATERIAL

Help Videos
To give more help for those who find learning from a book difficult we have placed some videos on our Youtube channels which deal with Viking era sword and shields. We have set up a special channel for Viking era material.
Our channels are called.
- Viking Guide Books
- Arts Of Mars Historical European Martial Arts

Find out more information at the following web site or sign up for our newsletter:
www.artsofmars.com

Watch out for our **online learning program** starting in 2014.

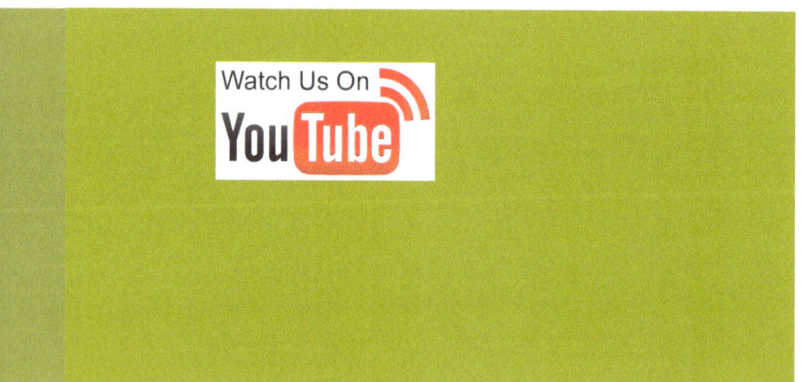

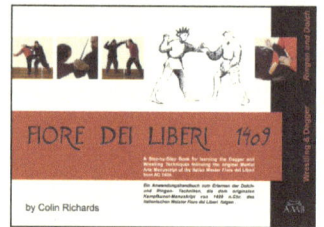

Fiore dei Liberi 1409
Wrestling & Dagger
Ringen & Dolch

Price: 44,95 Euro

This book covers the Wrestling and Dagger techniques of Fiore Dei Liberi from the 'Getty' version of the 'Fior di Battaglia'. Included is a selection of the 'Pisani-Dossi' 'Flos Duellatorum' dagger techniques. All techniques are described in both English and German languages. This is a step by step guide to the wrestling and dagger techniques of Fiore Dei Liberi using a new approach. Using a unique Timeline system, the photographs in the book detail the stages of each technique as they occur in time, with a separate close up focus on hand and foot movements, each positioned in the Timeline at the correct place. The whole book has been designed around the needs of the student who wishes to learn the actual techniques. This system allows the reader to follow the whole technique from start to finish and to learn it. This book is full colour and has approximately 800 pictures and 208 sides sewn, hard back, protected paper designed to survive the hard wear and tear of the training hall!

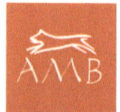

Books and DVDs by
Arts of Mars Books
Publishing House
Germany

All Books are available at **Swordexperts.com**

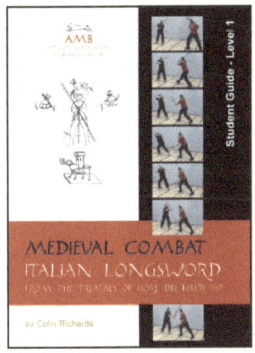

**Fiore dei Liberi 1409
Medieval Sword fighting
Student Guide Level 1**

Price: 39,90 Euro

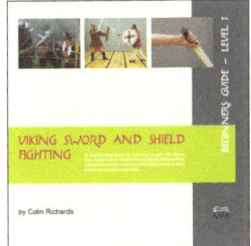

**Viking Sword
and Shield Fighting
Beginners Guide Level 1**

Price: 24,90 Euro

The Italian Martial Arts Master Fiore dei Liberi wrote his highly effective fighting techniques down for future generations to delve into the mysteries of the world of knightly combat. We present this valuable cultural heritage for those interested in historical combat in three DVDs, the first of which "Student Guide - Level 1" includes the following: Gripping the Sword, Breathing Technique, Stance Turning, Tactical Stepping, Basic Guard Positions, Cutting with the Sword, Thrusting with the Sword, Distance, Single Person Drills and Partner Drills! This DVD is a must for those who seriously want to learn the fundamental principles of Fiore dei Liberi's Longsword Combat System. This DVD is structured for easy learning for both single persons and groups and is finely tuned to help any experience level from absolute beginner to advanced practitioner.

This is a full colour step by step guide for beginners on how to fight safely with a Viking sword and shield. This book is useful for people interested in Stage Combat, Historical European Martial Arts and Re-enactors. It describes techniques, drills and common errors, in a simple but clear way using the unique Timeline system, so that people can follow each step easily and quickly. The author Colin Richards has 34 year experience in fighting with weapons and especially the Viking sword and shield combination. He has taught well over 2500 people in this combat art. The book also includes rules of engagement and a sample fight, and where to obtain good reliable equipment for this activity.

**Joachim Meyers
Kunst des Fechtens**

Price: 39,90 Euro

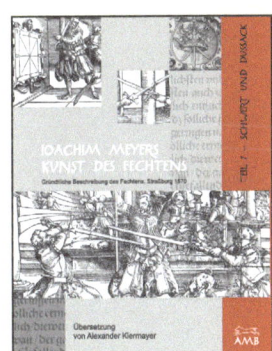

Joachim Meyer wrote an impressive text book on the state of German martial arts in the second half of the 16th Century. At the time in which it was printed, it was an important and pioneering work, for it was the first book of its kind, which was actually written for students of swordsmanship and described a systematic learning system. The author Alexander Kiermayer has transferred the work of Joachim Meyer in the modern German language and has processed it so that it is easily accessible for the modern reader. The original unique wood-cuts, are also included in the translation. To allow the reader an easier understanding of the text by Joachim Meyer, the corresponding relevant parts have been extracted from the woodcuts and arranged next to the descriptive text. Thus, the book includes within the 240 pages 189 illustrations from contemporary woodcuts, and graphics.

SWORD EXPERTS

**You
want to learn Historical European Martial Arts**

**We
have got the equipment!**

**Longswords • Single Handed Swords • Daggers
Fencing Masks • Gloves • Groin and Breast Protection
Throat Protection • Jackets
Books • DVD and more**

Supplied by
Arts of Mars Books
Allstar • Peter Regenyei • PBT • Purple Heart Armouries • Samurai Sports
Seelenschmiede • SPES • The Knightshop and more...

**Fast Delivery World Wide!
Best Price Guaranty!
High Quality Standard!
Top Offers!**

www.Swordexperts.com

www.ingramcontent.com/pod-product-compliance
Ingram Content Group UK Ltd.
Pitfield, Milton Keynes, MK11 3LW, UK
UKHW060138240426
12048UKWH00003B/85